Intimate Partner Violence: Risk and Vulnerability Factors, Health Promotion and Prevention in Educational and Healthcare Contexts

Intimate Partner Violence: Risk and Vulnerability Factors, Health Promotion and Prevention in Educational and Healthcare Contexts

Editors

Isabel Cuadrado-Gordillo
Guadalupe Martín-Mora Parra

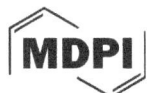

Basel • Beijing • Wuhan • Barcelona • Belgrade • Novi Sad • Cluj • Manchester

Editors
Isabel Cuadrado-Gordillo
Department of Psychology
Faculty of Education
and Psychology
University of Extremadura
Badajoz, Spain

Guadalupe Martín-Mora Parra
Department of Psychology
Faculty of Education
and Psychology
University of Extremadura
Badajoz, Spain

Editorial Office
MDPI
St. Alban-Anlage 66
4052 Basel, Switzerland

This is a reprint of articles from the Special Issue published online in the open access journal *Healthcare* (ISSN 2227-9032) (available at: https://www.mdpi.com/journal/healthcare/special_issues/195X5IW84N).

For citation purposes, cite each article independently as indicated on the article page online and as indicated below:

Lastname, A.A.; Lastname, B.B. Article Title. *Journal Name* **Year**, *Volume Number*, Page Range.

ISBN 978-3-0365-9522-1 (Hbk)
ISBN 978-3-0365-9523-8 (PDF)
doi.org/10.3390/books978-3-0365-9523-8

© 2023 by the authors. Articles in this book are Open Access and distributed under the Creative Commons Attribution (CC BY) license. The book as a whole is distributed by MDPI under the terms and conditions of the Creative Commons Attribution-NonCommercial-NoDerivs (CC BY-NC-ND) license.

Contents

About the Editors vii

Isabel Cuadrado-Gordillo, Guadalupe Martín-Mora-Parra and Ismael Puig-Amores
Victimization Perceived and Experienced by Teens in an Abusive Dating Relationship:
The Need to Tear down Social Myths
Reprinted from: *Healthcare* **2023**, *11*, 1639, doi:10.3390/healthcare11111639 1

**Allison Uvelli, Cristina Duranti, Giulia Salvo, Anna Coluccia, Giacomo Gualtieri and
Fabio Ferretti**
The Risk Factors of Chronic Pain in Victims of Violence: A Scoping Review
Reprinted from: *Healthcare* **2023**, *11*, 2421, doi:10.3390/healthcare11172421 15

**Noelia Aguilera-Jiménez, Luis Rodríguez-Franco, Francisco Javier Rodríguez-Díaz,
Jose Ramón Alameda-Bailén and Susana G. Paíno-Quesada**
Victimization and Perception of Abuse in Adolescent and Young Homosexual and Heterosexual
Couples in Spain
Reprinted from: *Healthcare* **2023**, *11*, 1873, doi:10.3390/healthcare11131873 31

Jayamini Chathurika Rathnayake, Nadirah Mat Pozian, Julie-Anne Carroll and Julie King
Barriers Faced by Australian and New Zealand Women When Sharing Experiences of Family
Violence with Primary Healthcare Providers: A Scoping Review
Reprinted from: *Healthcare* **2023**, *11*, 2486, doi:10.3390/healthcare11182486 49

Aisa Burgwal, Jara Van Wiele and Joz Motmans
The Impact of Sexual Violence on Quality of Life and Mental Wellbeing in Transgender and
Gender-Diverse Adolescents and Young Adults: A Mixed-Methods Approach
Reprinted from: *Healthcare* **2023**, *11*, 2281, doi:10.3390/healthcare11162281 63

Leonor Garay-Villarroel, Angela Castrechini-Trotta and Immaculada Armadans-Tremolosa
Risk Factors Linked to Violence in Female Same-Sex Couples in Hispanic America: A Scoping
Review
Reprinted from: *Healthcare* **2023**, *11*, 2456, doi:10.3390/healthcare11172456 79

María Pilar Salguero-Alcañiz, Ana Merchán-Clavellino and Jose Ramón Alameda-Bailén
Youth Dating Violence, Behavioral Sensitivity, and Emotional Intelligence: A Mediation
Analysis
Reprinted from: *Healthcare* **2023**, *11*, 2445, doi:10.3390/healthcare11172445 97

Xavier Calvet and Leonor M. Cantera
Prevalence and Characteristics of Sexual Victimization among Gay and Bisexual Men:
A Preliminary Study in Spain
Reprinted from: *Healthcare* **2023**, *11*, 2496, doi:10.3390/healthcare11182496 111

Nicolette Joh-Carnella, Eliza Livingston, Jill Stoddart and Barbara Fallon
Child Welfare Investigations of Exposure to Intimate Partner Violence Referred by Medical
Professionals in Ontario: A Uniquely Vulnerable Population?
Reprinted from: *Healthcare* **2023**, *11*, 2599, doi:10.3390/healthcare11182599 127

Claudia Sánchez and Cecilia Mota
Indicators Related to Marital Dissatisfaction
Reprinted from: *Healthcare* **2023**, *11*, 1959, doi:10.3390/healthcare11131959 137

About the Editors

Isabel Cuadrado-Gordillo

Isabel Cuadrado-Gordillo is a Developmental and Educational Psychology Professor and PhD tutor at the University of Extremadura, Spain. During her extent career, she has worked in multiple areas and has participated in many research projects, being the coordinator of the Educational Innovation and Research Group (GRIE). Her scientific interests include bullying and cyberbullying, dating violence, analysis of dialogic communication processes, and verbal and non-verbal discursive strategies. Professor Cuadrado-Gordillo has published numerous articles in international journals and books in scientific editorials. She has also edited Special Issues in international journals as a Guest Editor and has been on editorial boards and scientific committees for different conferences and congresses.

Guadalupe Martín-Mora Parra

Guadalupe Martín-Mora Parra is a Developmental and Educational Psychology Professor at the University of Extremadura, Spain. She is a member of the Educational Innovation and Research Group (GRIE), and her scientific interests include school violence, cyberbullying, dating violence, and communication in social networks. She has published articles in international journals, and some books. She has also collaborated as a Guest Editor in international journals.

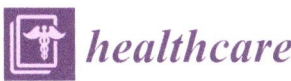 *healthcare*

Article

Victimization Perceived and Experienced by Teens in an Abusive Dating Relationship: The Need to Tear down Social Myths

Isabel Cuadrado-Gordillo *, Guadalupe Martín-Mora-Parra and Ismael Puig-Amores

Faculty of Education and Psychology, Department of Psychology and Anthropology, University of Extremadura, 06071 Badajoz, Spain; guadammp@gmail.com (G.M.-M.-P.); ipuigamores@unex.es (I.P.-A.)
* Correspondence: cuadrado@unex.es

Abstract: The phenomenon of adolescent dating violence is a social health problem that affects thousands of people in different contexts and parts of the world. To date, much of the work that has focused on analysing this phenomenon has tended to study it from the perspective of victimized adolescent girls, considering that gender violence predominates in violent pair relationships. Nonetheless, there is a growing body of evidence that the victimization of adolescent boys is a reality. Thus, mutual violence between boys and girls is increasingly prevalent. Given this context, the present study's objective was to analyse and compare the victimization profile of a sample of female and male adolescents, taking into account the variables most commonly associated with victimization in these abusive relationships (perceived violence suffered, perceived severity, sexism, and moral disengagement). With this objective, different instruments were administered (CUVINO, Scale of Detection of Sexism Adolescents (DSA), and Mechanism of Moral Disengagement Scale (MMDS)). Data analysis based on the construction of a multiple linear regression model confirmed that the boys and girls in the sample revealed having suffered violence from their partners to a different degree. It is evident that the victimization profile of the two sexes is different. Thus, boys show less perception of severity, more sexism, and greater use of certain moral disengagement mechanisms than girls. These results reveal the need to tear down social myths and construct prevention programs that take into account different victimization profiles.

Keywords: teen dating violence; male victimization; female victimization; moral disengagement; sexism

1. Introduction

Dating violence is one of the most common types of abuse among adolescents and young adults. These aggressions between dating couples begin at a very young age and can continue throughout life with different partners and relationships [1]. Thus, this phenomenon has been pointed to as one of the main factors associated with increased risks of abuse in adults [2].

The seriousness of the phenomenon has led to its global consideration as a social health problem of the first order and has encouraged the creation of various resources and programs for the care of victims, especially women. This fact highlights the general tendency to associate violence in pair relationships with the victimization of women. Gender violence based on control, abuse, and the development of asymmetric relationships is highly frequent throughout the world [3]. It has been pointed out that boys tend to show greater acceptance of violence within the couple [4], making it more likely that they become aggressors [5]. Nonetheless, neither the definition of adolescent dating violence nor that of violence in intimate relationships between adults is limited to gender violence.

The World Health Organization [6] and the Center for Disease Control and Prevention [7] establish violence in intimate relationships as being any conduct that causes the victim physical, psychological, or sexual harm, regardless of sex, gender, or the direction of aggressions [8]. With this, either member of the couple could in principle play the role of both victim and aggressor [9]. Evidence of male victimization in pair relationships has been found since the mid-1970s [10]. More recently, studies such as those of [11–15] have revealed victimization and bidirectional violence within the couple and a growing proportion of male victims [16], giving rise to different profiles of victimization and aggression in sentimental relationships.

There has been less research on male victimization than has been directed towards women. Some studies have pointed out, however, that men and women suffer similar attacks. For example, research conducted by the Spanish Government on violence in adolescent couples in 2015 revealed that both boys and girls tend to accept a certain degree of control by their partner [17], and this is also a common fact among adult couples [18,19]. Psychologists specialized in caring for adolescent girls victimized in a dating relationship point out that these young women often recognize that they perpetrate or have perpetrated aggression (especially control) towards their partners, largely copying the type of behaviour that boys display towards them [20].

However, control is not the only violent behaviour committed by female aggressors. It has been noted that girls' acceptance of violence is related to their own physical aggression towards their partners [21]. In a study carried out by Hines and Douglas [19], 77.5% of the sample of men reported having suffered minor physical attacks by their partner in the previous year, while 35.1% claimed to have suffered serious injuries. Recent studies have confirmed the presence of male victims of physical violence, but in different proportions [22,23]. Likewise, various works have pointed not only to the high prevalence of psychological violence in abusive relationships but also to the reciprocity and symmetry in the aggressions committed between men and women [18,24–27]. Similar conclusions were revealed by other studies, such as those carried out by Sears, Byers, and Price [28], who indicated that 35% of men and 47% of women confessed to having perpetrated psychological aggression towards their partners. With respect to addressing sexual violence, some studies have also pointed out that male victimization is a result of non-consensual sexual assaults by their partners [19,29]. In young adult and adolescent couples, research on male victimization and mutual aggression has been even less extensive, although various authors have revealed its existence in different contexts and countries [30–33]. Recently, some authors have reported similar results to those found among adult couples. Those workers indicate the existence of up to four different profiles of victimization and aggression, as well as the presence of reciprocal violence in young couples [34]. The first of these profiles involves low-intensity aggression towards an adolescent partner, directed at both boys (54%) and girls (40%). This study revealed the existence of mutual aggressions of psychological (34% girls and 33% boys) and physical (14% girls and 5% boys) types. The last profile found comprised multiple victimizations involving various types of violence in 8% of the cases of boys, with mutual psychological violence and sexual victimization being more prevalent among girls (12%).

Despite the evidence that has been found, there have been few studies that have analysed the specific profile of male victimization beyond merely pointing out its existence and the type of violence exerted or suffered. This fact further complicates the characterization and localization of factors that explain the initiation and maintenance of abuse in the case of boys. In contrast, the victimization of adolescent girls in this phenomenon has been widely studied, and they have been linked to such factors as the idealized vision of love [35] partly as a consequence of the great diffusion and consumption of audiovisual products of popular culture (film, television, and music) from early childhood onwards. The said ideal vision gives rise to the normalization, justification, and tolerance of aggression when it is committed by the partner [36] such that they understand violence as a normal way of interacting between couples, resulting in important consequences. This makes it hard for the victim to identify the victimization itself and ask for help. At the same time, other relevant factors linked to violence in adolescent couples have been noted. Examples are gender stereotypes and ambivalent sexism [37], the use of moral disengagement mechanisms as a means to justify the aggressor's conduct [38–40], the victim's inactivity to seek help [41], a history of domestic violence [4,42], and peer approval or personal factors such as negative emotionality [43].

Knowledge of the victimization profile of male adolescents is essential not only for reducing the taboo existing around the recognition and visibility of male victimization in dating relationships [22,44,45] but also for designing adequate prevention and care measures for not only women but also for men, resources that have up until now been neglected [46]. In this context, the principal objective of this study was (i) to investigate the victimization profile of adolescent boys in violent dating relationships, taking into account some of the factors traditionally linked to victimization (perception of severity in different types of violence, sexism, and moral disengagement); (ii) locate possible risk factors; and (iii) compare the profile found in victimized boys with that of victimized girls of the same age. This comparison is carried out to shed light on and help characterize male victimization and also to improve understanding of the phenomenon of dating violence and mutual aggression between men and women within the context of early intimate relationships.

2. Materials and Methods
2.1. Sample

The sample of this cross-sectional study comprised a total of 2577 adolescent students between the ages of 14 and 19 (44.8% boys). Participants were selected randomly and proportionally by a stratified sampling process in different stages. The process focused on randomly selecting a group of students that included different educational levels. Thus, the participants are students of lower secondary (ESO), upper secondary (Baccalaureate), and higher education (university and professional training). These students are from different areas of the Extremadura Region, including its two provinces (Cáceres and Badajoz), in the southwest of Spain. The selected areas cover both urban and rural zones of the region, with different socioeconomic characteristics and levels. Thus, approximately half of the sample belong to families exhibiting a medium–high level of purchasing power, and the other half exhibit a medium–low level of purchasing power. Similarly, the families had different academic levels, with half of the parents having completed higher education (Higher Level Education Cycles or University Studies) and the other half having completed secondary studies (Intermediate Training Cycles or Baccalaureate Certificate) or basic education.

In each of the schools selected, the questionnaires were administered collectively from the 3rd year of ESO to the 2nd year of Baccalaureate. The participants studying higher education were in their first year of university or the first year of their professional training. Their ages depended on their academic level (3rd ESO: 14–15 years; 4th ESO: 15–16 years; 1st Baccalaureate: 16–17 years; 2nd Baccalaureate: 17–18 years; university and 1st year of professional training: 18–19 years).

2.2. Instruments

Dating Violence Questionnaire, CUVINO [47]: This questionnaire has a total of 61 items, and they are grouped into two different blocks. The first addresses the types and incidences of violence that adolescents have received from their partners as well as the perception of severity they have regarding abusive behaviour. There are eight modalities of aggression considered for both frequency and perception of severity: detachment ("Is a good student, but is always late at meetings, does not fulfill his/her promises, and is irresponsible"), humiliation ("Ridicules your way of expressing yourself"), sexual ("You feel forced to perform certain sexual acts"), coercion (Threatens to commit suicide or hurt himself/herself if you leave him/her"), physical ("Has thrown blunt instruments at you"), gender ("Has ridiculed or insulted women or men as a group"), emotional punishment ("Refuses to give you support or affection as punishment"), and instrumental punishment ("Has stolen from you").

The first block uses a five-point anchor Likert-type scale with five anchor points ranging from "never" to "almost always". The reliability analysis (Cronbach's alpha) obtained from the sample of this study produced values ranging from 0.66 to 0.83 for the envisaged types. On the other hand, the perception of severity uses a five-point Likert-type scale with 1 being "a lot" and 5 being "not at all". The reliability for these modalities ranged from 0.71 to 0.84.

The second block focuses on victimization and the perception teenagers have of their characteristics as victims (duration of the relationship, attempts to break up, actual relationship with the aggressor, etc.).

Scale of Detection of Sexism in Adolescents (Escala de Detección de Sexismo en Adolescentes, DSA): This scale assesses the sexist attitudes that adolescents have towards traditional gender traits and roles, including two scales—hostile sexism and benevolent sexism [48]. Additionally, it has two secondary scales—sexist traits associated with F/M and the ability of each sex to perform roles and functions. The scale features six Likert-type points ranging from "totally disagree" to "totally agree". The reliability analysis (Cronbach's alpha) produced a value of 0.89 for the instrument overall, 0.91 for the hostile dimension, and 0.85 for the benevolent dimension.

Mechanisms of Moral Disengagement Scale (MMDS) [49]: This last questionnaire has a total of 32 items. These items allow obtaining 8 partial scores: moral justification, euphemistic language, advantageous comparison, displacement of responsibility, distortion of responsibility, distortion of consequences, attribution of blame, and dehumanization. The scale is a 5-anchor Likert-type scale ranging from "Strongly disagree" to "Strongly agree". The internal consistency of the test (Cronbach's alpha) is 0.74, and the reliability of the 8 mechanisms ranges between 0.72 and 0.81.

2.3. Procedure

Prior to the distribution of the questionnaires to the adolescents, both the research objectives and the procedure, instruments, and techniques used were checked and approved by the Bioethics and Biosafety Committee of the University of Extremadura (Spain) (Ref. 18/2017). The second step of the research study consisted in obtaining authorization from the Regional Educational Administration, and the project and its objectives were presented. Later, the management teams of lower and upper secondary schools were approached to invite them to participate in the study, describing the objectives and purpose of the study and the use of the data and ensuring the privacy and anonymity of adolescents. The written invitation was followed by personal telephone calls to the head teacher of each school to coordinate the collection of data covering the different levels (day and time of data collection).

Once authorizations to enter schools had been obtained, parental approval was also requested, considering that most participants were minors, by means of a document describing the nature of the study, the objectives, and the mechanisms used to guarantee the anonymity and confidentiality of the collected data. The letter was accompanied by an authorization form that parents had to sign and send back to the school in order to authorize the participation of their children in the study. In the case of participants of legal age (university students or professional training), the purpose of the study and its objectives were explained directly to them, ensuring the privacy and anonymity of responses. Additionally, they were asked to sign an informed consent document.

After obtaining authorization, the questionnaires were distributed in hard copies and completed by the participants. All questionnaires were completed collectively in each class and educational level. The instructions given by the researchers were the same in every class (anonymity was ensured, the Likert-scale was explained, the minimum time for a relationship (about a month), etc.). Additionally, we stayed in the class while the students filled out different questionnaires in order to clarify any possible doubts they could have.

2.4. Data Analysis

The data were analysed using statistical software package SPSS vn 24. Preliminary analyses began with the identification of victimized adolescents. Subjects who scored 0 on the CUVINO questionnaire were considered non-victims of adolescent dating violence. Those who scored higher than 0 were considered victims and assigned to two different victimization groups based on the frequency with which they had undergone the attacks: those who scored less than 3 were assigned to the "Sometimes" victim of violence group, and those with scores greater than 3 were classified as "Frequent" victims.

Secondly, the incidence of perceived violence suffered, the perception of the severity of the violent behaviours, the degree of sexism (hostile sexism, benevolent sexism, sexist trait, and sexist attitude), and the use of moral disengagement mechanisms (moral justification, euphemistic language, advantageous comparison, displacement of responsibility, distortion of consequences, attribution of blame, and dehumanization) were determined. The descriptive statistics of the study variables were computed, and Student's t-test was used to compare each dimension by sex. The strength of the associations was measured using Cramér's V and the chi-squared test.

Finally, the variables associated with the risk of violence were analysed by means of stepwise multiple linear regression, and these included the total score obtained with respect to violence as the dependent variable; the sex of the victims and different dimensions of the scales used during data acquisition (perceived severity of violent behaviour, sexism, and moral disengagement mechanisms) were used as predictor variables.

3. Results

The preliminary analyses revealed that, of the total sample of 2577 adolescents, 1232 had suffered violence on some occasions. Of these, 1190 adolescents are classified as victims who have suffered dating violence "sometimes" (sometimes frequently in CUVINO), and 42 perceive themselves as "frequent" victims (usually almost always in CUVINO); thus, the number of victims decreases as the frequency of violence increases. In both groups, the number of female adolescent victims is greater (Table 1).

Table 1. Victimized adolescents.

	Sometimes	Frequently	Total
Male	500	18	518
Female	690	24	714
Total	1190	42	1232

The analysis of the CUVINO questionnaire, which directly asks the participants if they have ever felt mistreated (item 45), shows that, despite the fact that boys and girls indicate having suffered violence to a different extent, only 22 boys identify themselves as victims of abuse, while 69 girls report having been mistreated in a dating relationship.

With respect to the types of violence suffered, male and female victims coincide in that the most prevalent types are detachment, coercion, and emotional punishment. The analysis of associations between the variables, as measured using the chi-squared and Cramér's V statistics, reveals that there is a statistically significant relationship between the sex of the victims and coercion incidence ($\chi^2 = 39.91$; $V = 0.180$; $p < 0.01$), emotional punishment incidence ($\chi^2 = 38.242$; $V = 0.176$; $p < 0.001$), and instrumental punishment incidence ($\chi^2 = 21.49$; $V = 0.132$; $p < 0.01$) (Table 2). Thus, although the three most frequent types of violence are identical in male and female victims, boys perceive a greater degree of violence suffered in these three types of abuse.

With regard to the victims' perception of the severity of different types of violence, there are differences in the aggression that boys and girls consider as most serious. Specifically, boys point to physical violence severity (X = 4.10; SD = 1.19), humiliation severity (X = 4.06; SD = 1.19), and instrumental punishment severity (X = 4.04; SD = 1.16), and girls point to physical violence severity (X = 4.62; SD = 0.89), humiliation severity (X = 4.50; SD = 0.79), and sexual violence severity (X = 4.49; SD = 0.84). Likewise, the analysis of associations between the variables using the chi-squared statistic shows a statistically significant association between the perception of severity with respect to all types of violence and the victim's sex. Being male or female is linked to the importance given to different types of violence, with the latter perceiving greater severity in all types of analysed victimization.

Table 2. Statistical description of the CUVINO questionnaire.

	Male Victims		Female Victims			
	$\bar{x}$	SD	$\bar{x}$	SD	χ^2	V
Detachment incidence	1.52	0.54	1.53	0.55	28.54	0.152
Humiliation incidence	1.25	0.38	1.23	0.38	10.73	0.093
Sexual incidence	1.23	0.44	1.19	0.40	18.79	0.124
Coercion incidence	1.43	0.46	1.39	0.53	39.91 **	0.180 **
Physical incidence	1.13	0.35	1.1	0.27	23.55	0.138
Gender incidence	1.22	0.35	1.25	0.50	16.98	0.117
Emotional Punishment incidence	1.41	0.55	1.31	0.51	38.242 ***	0.176 ***
Instrumental Punishment incidence	1.11	0.37	1.05	0.20	21.49 **	0.132 **
Detachment severity	3.61	0.97	4.35	0.71	199.00 ***	0.406 ***
Humiliation severity	4.06	1.19	4.50	0.79	223.86 ***	0.432 ***
Sexual severity	3.62	1.18	4.49	0.84	474.75 ***	0.630 ***
Coercion severity	3.62	0.97	4.25	0.81	219.14 ***	0.425 ***
Physical severity	4.10	1.19	4.62	0.89	198.33 ***	0.407 ***
Gender severity	3.62	1.18	4.41	0.84	272.73 ***	0.477 ***
Emotional Punishment severity	3.47	1.07	4.13	0.95	149.78 ***	0.353 ***
Instrumental Punishment severity	4.04	1.16	4.43	0.95	97.60 ***	0.286 ***

** $p < 0.01$; *** $p < 0.001$.

The results of the sexism questionnaire show differences between the degree of sexism of male victims and female victims in the four analysed variables. Adolescent girls score lower than boys on the four subscales, thus showing a lesser degree of sexism than boys. This fact is especially significant in the case of hostile sexism and the attitude that the participants show towards the capacity of men and women to carry out different roles and social functions. In this sense, an association is found between the sex of adolescent victims and the dimensions "hostile sexism" ($\chi^2 = 0.37. p < 0.001$) and "attitude towards performance of roles and functions" ($\chi^2 = 0.36; p < 0.001$) (Table 3).

Table 3. Descriptive analysis sexism questionnaire.

	Male Victims		Female Victims			
	$\bar{x}$	SD	$\bar{x}$	SD	χ^2	V
Hostile sexism	1.61	0.72	1.35	0.64	167.463 ***	0.37 ***
Benevolent sexism	2.30	0.89	2.29	0.98	59.454	0.22
Sexist traits associated with F/M	2.10	0.78	2.07	0.84	70.725	0.24
Ability of each sex to perform roles and functions	1.60	0.75	1.33	0.65	156.573 ***	0.36 ***

*** $p < 0.001$.

The analysis of the moral disengagement scale once again points to differences in the use that boys and girls make of these mechanisms. Thus, descriptive statistics reveal that the resources most used by boys are "moral justification" (X = 2.01; SD = 0.55), "advantageous comparison" (X = 1.63; SD = 0.49), and "displacement of responsibility" (X = 1.59; SD = 0.46). The victimized adolescent girls, to a greater extent, used "moral justification" (X = 1.68; SD = 0.45), "displacement of responsibility" (X = 1.55; SD = 0.43), and "advantageous comparison" (X = 1.44; SD = 0.38). Hence, while they use the same mechanisms, their relative importance is different, with victimized boys also indicating a higher frequency of use. In sum, there is a statistically significant association between the sex of the victims and the use of the seven moral disengagement mechanisms (Table 4).

Table 4. Descriptive analysis moral disengagement questionnaire.

	Male Victims		Female Victims			
	$\bar{x}$	SD	$\bar{x}$	SD	χ^2	V
Moral justification	2.01	0.55	1.68	0.45	142.63 ***	0.342 ***
Euphemistic language	1.37	0.38	1.16	0.28	131.72 ***	0.329 ***
Advantageous comparison	1.63	0.49	1.44	0.38	63.18 ***	0.228 ***
Diffusion of responsability	1.59	0.46	1.55	0.43	16.23 **	0.115
Distorsión of consequences	1.42	0.37	1.28	0.29	52.829 ***	0.208 ***
Ascription of blame	1.52	0.40	1.38	0.34	58.759 ***	0.220 ***
Dehumanization	1.53	0.50	1.33	0.40	82.414 ***	0.260 ***

** $p < 0.01$; *** $p < 0.001$.

To determine whether there are differences by sex in the study's variables, an analysis of differences was performed using Student's t-test (Table 5). There were statistically significant differences in the factors "perception of severity" ($t_{1015.358} = -13.31$; $p < 0.001$), "hostile sexism" ($t_{1072.025} = 6.39$; $p < 0.001$), "attitude of each sex to performance of roles" ($t_{1040.804} = 6.42$; $p < 0.001$), "moral justification" ($t_{1032.755} = 12.01$; $p < 0.001$), "euphemistic language" ($t_{894.995} = 10.44$; $p < 0.001$), "advantageous comparison" ($t_{1031.426} = 6.95$; $p < 0.001$), " diffusion of responsibility" ($t_{1045.414} = 2.22$; $p < 0.05$), "distortion of consequences" ($t_{900.854} = 6.49$; $p < 0.001$), "victim blaming" ($t_{966.027} = 7.22$; $p < 0.001$), and "dehumanization" ($t_{962.802} = 7.77$; $p < 0.001$).

Table 5. Analysis of mean differences.

	T	gl	p	Mean Differences
Total violence incidence	1.76	1097.543	0.08	0.03
Total perception of severity	13.31	1015.358	0.000	0.73
Hostile sexism	6.39	1072.025	0.000	0.26
Benevolent sexism	0.25	1174.757	0.79	0.01
Sexist traits associated with F/M	0.013	1179.845	0.99	0.06
Attitudes of each sex to performance of roles	6.42	1040.804	0.000	0.30
Moral justification	12.01	1032.755	0.000	0.34
Euphemistic language	10.44	894.995	0.000	0.22
Advantageous comparison	6.95	1031.426	0.000	0.17
Diffusion of responsability	2.22	1045.414	0.02	0.06
Distorsión of consequences	6.49	900.854	0.000	0.13
Victims blaming	7.22	966.027	0.000	0.15
Dehumanization	7.77	962.802	0.000	0.21

For the factor "negative perception of severity", the girls' mean scores are higher than the boys', but for all moral disengagement mechanisms, the contrary is the case. Nonetheless, the calculated effect sizes for most constructs are very small (<0.20). The exceptions are "perception of severity", "hostile sexism", "fitness of each sex to perform roles and functions", "moral justification", "euphemistic language", and "dehumanization" (moderate effect sizes between 0.20 and 0.70). It could be considered that, although significant, the contribution is not relevant in the rest of the variables.

Finally, stepwise multiple linear regression was used to analyse the variables that were associated with the perceived violence suffered. The dependent variable was the perceived violence suffered. The predictor variables were the dimensions of the administered scales (perception of severity with respect to the different types of violence, hostile sexism, benevolent sexism, sexist attitude, sexist trait, and moral disengagement mechanisms), adding the sex of the participants and the age as control variables in order to eliminate its effect from the model. The resultant models had no problems with respect to multicollinearity (VIF < 5), and the percentages of variance explained ranged from 10% to 11%.

Table 6 lists the results of the two models. In Model 1, the male victims' perceived violence that they have suffered is predicted, to the greatest extent, by annoyance with the "humiliation" type of violence. In Model 2, the female victims' perceived violence that they have suffered is predicted to the greatest extent by annoyance with the "instrumental punishment" type of violence (Table 6).

Table 6. Linear regression.

	Model 1: Male		R	R^2	F		Model 2: Female		R	R^2	F
1	Hostile sexism	0.205 ***	0.042	0.040	21.455	1	Instrumental violence severity	−0.221 ***	0.049	0.047	34.847
2	Hostile sexism	0.177 ***	0.068	0.065	17.864	2	Instrumental violence severity	−0.211 ***	0.084	0.081	31.137
	Negative emotions	0.164 ***					Negative emotions	0.188 ***			
3	Hostile sexism	0.148 ***	0.079	0.073	13.863	3	Instrumental violence severity	−0.340 ***	0.098	0.094	24.583
	Negative emotions	0.166 ***					Negative emotions	−191 ***			
	Instrumental violence severity	−0.106 *					Detachment severity	0.176 ***			
4	Hostile sexism	0.162 ***	0.092	0.085	12.302	4	Instrumental violence severity	−0.340 ***	0.11	0.105	20.915
	Negative emotions	0.158 ***					Negative emotions	0.161 ***			
	Instrumental violence severity	−0.236 ***					Detachment severity	0.184 ***			
	Detachment severity	0.177 ***					Moral justification	0.114 **			
5	Hostile sexism	0.163 ***	0.11	0.096	11.327						
	Negative emotions	0.157 ***									
	Instrumental violence severity	−0.138 *									
	Detachment severity	0.295 ***									
	Humiliation severity	−0.232 **									
6	Hostile sexism	0.172 ***	0.12	0.104	10.424						
	Negative emotions	0.153 ***									
	Instrumental violence severity	−0.170 *									
	Detachment severity	0.242 **									
	Humiliation severity	−0.339 ***									
	Coercion severity	0.209 *									

* $p < 0.05$; ** $p < 0.01$; *** $p < 0.001$.

4. Discussion

The results found in this study reveal the high presence of victimization in adolescent dating relationships, with both boys and girls being subjected to victimization. Thus, it was observed that the violence suffered in the first dating relationship, far from being confined to women, equally affects young men. Adolescent boys suffer abuse in their romantic relationships both sporadically and frequently, similarly to what was found in relation to female victimization. This fact seems to point to the high prevalence of mutual violence in abusive relationships, following the same pattern as found in recent research with adults [50]. With this, victimization in adolescent dating would not only be one of the main factors that predict violence between adult couples but would also be one of the main predictors of reciprocal violence in such relationships.

In contrast, the results reveal that boys show a lower degree of perception of severity than girls in all the types of analysed violence. While the girls perceive violence as serious, the boys show less rejection of abuse, downplaying violent behaviour to a certain extent. In relation to this, various studies [51,52] have shown that men who tend to accept violence are those who also tend to commit more acts of abuse towards their partner, thus adopting the role of the aggressor more easily. Nonetheless, this acceptance of dating violence could also cause boys, even when they are the ones who suffer from this type of violent behaviour, to view it as less important.

Based on the above, there is a fundamental difference between adolescent boys and girls victimized in a relationship. While girls normalize the violence perpetrated by their partners as being a result of factors such as the idealization of love [53] or the presence of latent benevolent sexism [37], they continue to be aware of the seriousness of the abuses even when they have normalized them [54]. With this, it is possible that prevention campaigns and public health interventions that are focused on the empowerment of women and on the modification of the structural environment of women [55], by highlighting the undesirability of violence, have had a positive effect on pair relationships. They seem to have failed, however, to get young women to identify their own victimization, ultimately prolonging the maintenance of violence in dating [56].

Boys may also accept violence, but for different reasons. In this sense, various authors have pointed to the taboo existing in society regarding the consideration of men as victims [22,44,45]. This fact may encourage mistreated adolescent boys to avoid interpreting the violence they receive as abuse, thus refusing to see themselves as victims. This may be of great importance to them with respect to protecting their self-esteem, but at the same time, it would prolong their victimization and their maintenance of the violent dating relationship. Additionally, it is possible that, from a masculine perspective, the abuses are classified as normal forms of relating to the partner, and the importance of the different types of abuse and aggressive behaviours is interpreted as being less serious. In this regard, it has been found that violence is better tolerated by men when the aggressors are women [57]. Likewise, some studies have found that supporting a patriarchal ideology, with the assumption of male and female stereotypes and sexual roles, encourages the growth of violence in pair relationships [58] and resistance to an awareness of victimization behaviours. These findings point in the same direction as the results of this present study: i.e., that adolescent boys present a greater degree of hostile sexism and sexist attitudes than girls. Both types of sexism seem to support the acceptance of violence within couples, especially for young men and women who tend to adopt the stereotype associated with their gender role.

While, according to the analysis of results, hostile sexism and sexist attitudes are associated with victimized boys, benevolent sexism appears in all victims regardless of their sex. These findings reinforce the presence of a high degree of normalization of certain types of violence in the sense that girls believe that they must be protected by men [59] while simultaneously romanticizing and tolerating this type of behaviour with the belief that it is carried with the aim of caring for them. The boys, for their part, would adopt this role of protector, thinking that they exhibit behaviours that are not classified as abusive because they fit the stereotype of the man as a caregiver [60].

The belief that women need affection and the assumption that, to be happy, every man needs a woman could create a form of sexism directed towards men and women that, although seemingly contradictory, would actually be interdependent and complementary [61]. Then, without being aware of it, the victimized adolescent boys might also be taking on the hostile sexist stereotypes of women as being weak and inferior [62] to justify girls' violence, additionally believing that women do not have the capacity or ability to cause real harm with their violent behaviours.

Another relevant finding of the study is that victimized boys use moral disengagement mechanisms to a greater extent than girls. Other work too has suggested the existence of a consistent relationship between aggression and moral disengagement from the committed abuses [63]. Nonetheless, it seems that the use of these mechanisms is also important from the victim's perspective. In the case of boys, this finding of a greater frequency of use may be linked to a twofold objective. One is that possible aggressions committed in the context of a dating relationship are justified as a form of achieving personal objectives [64] within that relationship. The other is that these mechanisms would also fulfil the function of justifying both the individual's own position as a victim as well as the abuses perpetrated by their aggressors. The process followed would thus be similar to the justification that victims of bullying in school make with respect to the violent behaviour of their aggressors [65].

For their part, victimized girls might not need these moral disengagement tools to the same extent since they are already normalizing the violence; they normalize these situations as benevolent sexism and normalize violence via the use of the factors mentioned above. In this context, moral disengagement would be one more instrument combined with the rest of the factors that sustain victimization in the long term. The aggressions that girls commit towards their partners would not have such a marked need for moral justification since girls might see them as a right that they have in a social context of false empowerment [65,66], which places women in the same position as men. In this way, adolescent girls seem to tend to repeat the same type of maladjusted behaviour that they see in their aggressive partners, and this is a factor that fosters an increase in mutual aggression in adolescent dating relationships [20]. Similar results have been suggested in the contexts of bullying and cyberbullying in which victims of school violence tend to become aggressors in cyberspace, understanding these behaviours as a fully justified form of revenge [67–69] that provides some degree of compensation [70].

Differences that are found between the predictive models of the frequency of violence in boys and girls stand out. Firstly, the sex of the victim is not an important predictor variable. This reinforces the aforementioned idea of the great presence of mutual violence in adolescent dating relationships [30–34]. Then, there is the fact that although the boys share some of the same predictor variables with victimized girls, the model resulting for them includes a greater number of variables. The prediction of violence in the case of victimized boys includes variables such as hostile sexism and the perception of the severity of two specific and interrelated types of violence—humiliation and coercion. This fact is important, especially given that humiliation has been pointed out as a particularly serious type of abuse for men [71] due to its relationship with the social idea of masculinity [72]. Thus, authors such as those who published [73] have noted that men who feel they have been humiliated tend to respond violently to restore balance and preserve their reputation [74,75]. In recent studies, authors such as [71] have suggested the importance of deconstructing social myths around masculinity in order to prevent violent behaviour from being used as a means to demonstrate manhood. Thus, the assaults and abuse related to this specific type of violence might not only increase the victimization of boys in dating relationships but also foster a proportional increase in mutual aggression when the two partners try to restore balance, thus creating a downward spiral of abuse that teenage boys and girls find hard to escape.

On the contrary, in the case of girls, the regression model shows how the most important factor in predicting victimization is annoyance with the "instrumental punishment" type of violence. This finding could be related to the ideal vision of love, which increases the normalization, justification, and tolerance of aggression when it is committed by a partner [36]. This fact seems also to be linked with the use of moral justification as a tool to ignore abusive behavior [38–40].

5. Limitations

The study has some limitations that must be considered. First, it is cross-sectional. A longitudinal study could provide data on adolescents' evolution and the possible changes that might arise in aggressive dating relationships. Such data would help delve deeper into the evolution and development of victimized adolescents and make it possible to identify additional variables to take into account that would undoubtedly be of interest in the design of short-, medium-, and long-term prevention programs. Likewise, a possible future line of research would be to incorporate the virtual context into studies of the phenomenon of violence in adolescent dating. As digital natives, a large proportion of the abusive control behaviours that boys and girls exhibit are carried out using instant messaging applications and social networks. An in-depth analysis of these behaviours would help contextualize the phenomenon within today's information and communication society.

6. Conclusions

Teen dating violence has been studied extensively, but the field of adolescent male victimization has been less explored. The main contribution of the present study is its focus on male victims in an attempt to gain a broad and full understanding of the phenomenon. One of the main findings is that although boys perceive suffering different types of violence in their dating relationships, their perception of the severity of all types of analysed abuse is significantly lower than that indicated by female victims. In this way, the results show that boys give less importance to abuse than girls, even when they themselves are the victims. Nonetheless, neither boys nor girls seem to recognize their own victimization, leading to normalization and tolerance of violence that are motivated by different factors.

Other relevant findings indicate that boys present certain types of sexism more and exhibit a greater use of moral disengagement mechanisms than girls. The study thus reveals the importance of considering the sexism of victimized adolescents as an interdependent factor; in this case, the stereotypes that boys accept as their own encourage the stereotypes and roles that girls accept. Likewise, the use of moral disengagement mechanisms seems to have become another tool at the service of normalizing, justifying, and tolerating mutual violence in abusive relationships during adolescence. These discoveries have important practical applications. There is a need to put forward multidisciplinary strategies of prevention and intervention that are adapted to the characteristics of victims, and they should include boys in these interventions not only as possible aggressors but also as victims while considering the influence of cultural and social factors as well. Reciprocal violence needs to be recognized as a common problem in the phenomenon of adolescent dating violence.

Author Contributions: I.C.-G., G.M.-M.-P. and I.P.-A. contributed to the design, writing, and supervision of the article. All authors have read and agreed to the published version of the manuscript.

Funding: This research was funded by the Extremadura Government (Junta de Extremadura) and Feder Funds, grant number IB16011.

Institutional Review Board Statement: The study was conducted according to the guidelines of the Declaration of Helsinki and approved by the Bioethics and Biosafety Committee of the University of Extremadura (Spain) (Ref. 18/2017).

Informed Consent Statement: Informed consent was obtained from all subjects involved in the study.

Data Availability Statement: Data not available due to privacy.

Conflicts of Interest: The authors declare no conflict of interest.

References

1. Makepeace, J.M. Courtship violence among college students. *Fam. Relat.* **1981**, *30*, 97–102. [CrossRef]
2. Meneghel, S.N.; Portella, A.P. Femicides: Concepts, types and scenarios. *Ciência Saúde Coletiva* **2017**, *22*, 3077–3086. [CrossRef] [PubMed]
3. Ruiz-Pérez, I.; Pastor-Moreno, G. Measures to contain gender-based violence during the COVID-19 pandemic. *Gac. Sanit.* **2021**, *35*, 389–394. Available online: https://www.sciencedirect.com/science/article/pii/S0213911120300881 (accessed on 17 January 2023). [CrossRef]
4. Karlsson, M.E.; Temple, J.R.; Weston, R.; Le, V.D. Witnessing interparental violence and acceptance of dating violence as predictors for teen dating violence victimization. *Violence Against Women* **2016**, *22*, 625–646. [CrossRef] [PubMed]
5. Cauffman, E.; Feldman, S.S.; Jensen, L.A.; Arnett, J.J. The (un) acceptability of violence against peers and dates. *J. Adolesc. Res.* **2000**, *15*, 652–673. [CrossRef]
6. World Health Organization Violence against Women. Available online: http://www.who.int/news-room/fact-sheets/detail/violence-against-women (accessed on 17 January 2023).
7. Centers for Disease Control and Prevention. Intimate Partner Violence: Risk and Protective Factors. 2017. Available online: https://www.cdc.gov/violenceprevention/intimatepartnerviolence/riskprotectivefactors.html (accessed on 17 January 2023).
8. Jennings, W.G.; Okeem, C.; Piquero, A.R.; Sellers, C.S.; Theobald, D.; Farrington, D.P. Dating and intimate partner violence among young persons ages 15–30: Evidence from a systematic review. *Aggress. Violent Behav.* **2017**, *33*, 107–125. [CrossRef]
9. Rojas-Solís, J.L.; Guzmán-Pimentel, M.; Jiménez-Castro, M.P.; Martínez-Ruiz, L.; Flores-Hernández, B.G. La violencia hacia los hombres en la pareja heterosexual: Una revisión de revisiones. *Cienc. Y Soc.* **2019**, *44*, 57–70. [CrossRef]
10. Gelles, R.J. *The Violent Home: A Study of Physical Aggression between Husbands and Wives*; Sage: Beverly Hills, CA, USA, 1974.
11. Kumar, R. Domestic violence and mental health. *Delhi Psychiatry J.* **2012**, *15*, 274–278.
12. Barber, C.F. Domestic violence against men. *Nurs. Stand.* **2008**, *22*, 35. [CrossRef]
13. Holtzworth-Munroe, A. Male versus female intimate partner violence: Putting controversial findings into context. *J. Marriage Fam.* **2005**, *67*, 1120–1125. [CrossRef]
14. Tsang, W.W.H. Do male victims of intimate partner violence (IPV) deserve help? Some reflections based on a systematic review. *Hong Kong J. Soc. Work* **2015**, *49*, 51–63. [CrossRef]
15. Simon, C.T.; Tsang, W.H.W. Disclosure of victimization experiences of Chinese male survivors of intimate partner abuse. *Qual. Soc. Work.* **2018**, *17*, 744–761. [CrossRef]
16. Shuler, C.A. Male victims of intimate partner violence in the United States: An examination of the review of literature through the critical theoretical perspective. *Int. J. Crim. Justice Sci.* **2010**, *5*, 163.
17. Delegación del Gobierno para la Violencia de Género. La delegación del Gobierno para la Violencia de Género informa. Available online: https://violenciagenero.igualdad.gob.es/laDelegacionInforma/pdfs/DGVG_Informa_Macroencuesta_2015.pdf (accessed on 23 February 2023).
18. Laroche, D. *Aspects of the Context and Consequences of Domestic Violence*; desLibris: Ottawa, ON, Canada, 2005.
19. Hines, D.A.; Douglas, E.M. Sexual aggression experiences among male victims of physical partner violence: Prevalence, severity, and health correlates for male victims and their children. *Arch. Sex. Behav.* **2016**, *45*, 1133–1151. [CrossRef] [PubMed]
20. Cuadrado-Gordillo, I.; Martín-Mora-Parra, G.; Puig-Amores, I. Analysis of representations of the aid that public psychological support points provide to adolescent female victims of gender-based violence: Reformulation of policies and practices. *Int. J. Environ. Res. Public Health* **2022**, *19*, 8422. [CrossRef]
21. Ali, T.S.; Asad, N.; Mogren, I.; Krantz, G. Intimate partner violence in urban Pakistan: Prevalence, frequency, and risk factors. *Int. J. Womens Health* **2011**, *2011*, 111–115. [CrossRef]
22. Allen, E.; Bradley, M.S. Perceptions of harm, criminality, and law enforcement response: Comparing violence by men against women and violence by women against men. *Vict. Offender* **2018**, *13*, 373–389. [CrossRef]
23. Khan, A.R.; Arendse, N. Female perpetrated domestic violence against men and the case for Bangladesh. *J. Hum. Behav. Soc. Environ.* **2022**, *32*, 519–533. [CrossRef]
24. Black, M.C.; Basile, K.C.; Breiding, M.J.; Smith, S.G.; Walters, M.L.; Merrick, M.T.; Chen, J.; Stevens, M.R. *The National Intimate Partner and Sexual Violence Survey (NISVS): 2010 Summary Report*; National Center for Injury Prevention and Control, Centers for Disease Control and Prevention: Atlanta, GA, USA, 2011.
25. Breiding, M.J.; Chen, J.; Black, M.C. *Intimate Partner Violence in the United States—2010*; National Center for Injury Prevention and Control, Centers for Disease Control and Prevention: Atlanta, GA, USA, 2014.
26. Carney, M.M.; Barner, J.R. Prevalence of partner abuse: Rates of emotional abuse and control. *Partn. Abus.* **2012**, *3*, 286–335. [CrossRef]
27. Rey-Anacona, C.A. Prevalencia y tipos de maltrato en el noviazgo en adolescentes y adultos jóvenes. *Ter. Psicol.* **2013**, *31*, 143–154. [CrossRef]

28. Sears, H.; Byers, S.; Price, L. The co-occurrence of adolescent boys' and girls' use of psychologically, physically, and sexually abusive behaviours in their dating relationships. *J. Adolesc.* **2007**, *30*, 487–504. [CrossRef]
29. Weare, S. From coercion to physical force: Aggressive strategies used by women against men in "forced-to-penetrate" cases in the UK. *Arch. Sex. Behav.* **2018**, *47*, 2191–2205. [CrossRef]
30. Chiodo, D.; Crooks, C.V.; Wolfe, D.A.; McIsaac, C.; Hughes, R.; Jaffe, P.G. Longitudinal prediction and concurrent functioning of adolescent girls demonstrating various profiles of dating violence and victimization. *Prev. Sci.* **2012**, *13*, 350–359. [CrossRef] [PubMed]
31. Giordano, P.C.; Soto, D.A.; Manning, W.D.; Longmore, M.A. The characteristics of romantic relationships associated with teen dating violence. *Soc. Sci. Res.* **2010**, *39*, 863–874. [CrossRef] [PubMed]
32. Leal, F.; Reinoso, L.; Rojas, K.; Romero, R. Violencia en las relaciones de pareja en adolescentes escolares de Arica. *Rev. Infanc. Y Educ.* **2011**, *1*, 18–35.
33. Straus, M.A.; Mickey, E.L. Reliability, validity, and prevalence of partner violence measured by the conflict tactics scales in male-dominant nations. *Aggress. Violent Behav.* **2012**, *17*, 463–474. [CrossRef]
34. Théorêt, V.; Hébert, M.; Fernet, M.; Blais, M. Gender-specific patterns of teen dating violence in heterosexual relationships and their associations with attachment insecurities and emotion dysregulation. *J. Youth Adolesc.* **2021**, *50*, 246–259. [CrossRef]
35. Sanpedro, P. El mito del amor y sus consecuencias en los vínculos de pareja. *Disenso* **2005**, *45*, 5–20.
36. González, R.; Santana, J.D. La violencia en parejas jóvenes. *Psicothema* **2001**, *13*, 127–131.
37. Fernández-Antelo, I.; Cuadrado-Gordillo, I.; Martín-Mora Parra, G. Synergy between acceptance of violence and sexist attitudes as a dating violence risk factor. *Int. J. Environ. Res. Public Health* **2020**, *17*, 5209. [CrossRef]
38. Bandura, A. *Social Foundations of thought and Action*; Prentice-Hall: Englewood Cliffs, NJ, USA, 1986.
39. Tata, J. She said, he said. The influence of remedial accounts on third-party judgments of coworker sexualn harassment. *J. Manag.* **2000**, *26*, 1133–1156.
40. Quinn, B.A. Sexual harassment and masculinity: The power and meaning of "girl watching". *Gend. Soc.* **2002**, *16*, 386–402. [CrossRef]
41. Cuadrado-Gordillo, I.; Fernández-Antelo, I.; Martín-Mora Parra, G. Moral disengagement as a moderating factor in the relationship between the perception of dating violence and victimization. *Int. J. Environ. Res. Public Health* **2020**, *17*, 5164. [CrossRef] [PubMed]
42. Cascardi, M. From violence in the home to physical dating violence victimization: The mediating role of psychological distress in a prospective study of female adolescents. *J. Youth Adolesc.* **2016**, *45*, 777–792. [CrossRef]
43. Cuadrado-Gordillo, I.; Fernández-Antelo, I.; Martín-Mora Parra, G. Search for the profile of the victim of adolescent dating violence: An intersection of cognitive, emotional, and behavioral variables. *Int. J. Environ. Res. Public Health* **2020**, *17*, 8004. [CrossRef] [PubMed]
44. Espinoza, R.C.; Warner, D. Where do we go from here?: Examining intimate partner violence by bringing male victims, female perpetrators, and psychological sciences into the fold. *J. Fam. Violence* **2016**, *31*, 959–966. [CrossRef]
45. Navarro Ceja, N.; Salguero Velázquez, M.A.; Torres Velázquez, L.E.; Figueroa Perea, J.G. Voces silenciadas: Hombres que viven violencia en la relación de pareja. *La Ventana Rev. Estud. Género* **2019**, *6*, 136–172. [CrossRef]
46. Bates, E.A. Current controversies within intimate partner violence: Overlooking bidirectional violence. *J. Fam. Violence* **2016**, *31*, 937–940. [CrossRef]
47. Rodríguez-Franco, L.; Antuña, M.A.; Rodríguez-Díaz, F.J.; Herrero, F.J.; Nieves, V.E. Violencia de género en relaciones de pareja durante la adolescencia: Análisis diferencial del Cuestionario de Violencia entre Novios (CuViNo). In *Psicología Jurídica. Violencia y Víctimas*; Arce, R., Fariña, F., Alfaro, E., Civera, C., Tortosa, F., Eds.; Diputación de Valencia: Valencia, FL, USA, 2007; pp. 137–147.
48. Recio, P.; Cuadrado, I.; Ramos, E. Propiedades psicométricas de la Escala de Detección de Sexismo en Adolescentes (DSA). *Psicothema* **2007**, *19*, 522–528.
49. Bandura, A.; Barbaranelli, C.; Caprara, G.V.; Pastorelli, C. Mechanisms of moral disengagement in the exercise of moral agency. *J. Pers. Soc. Psychol.* **1996**, *71*, 364. [CrossRef]
50. Hine, B.; Noku, L.; Bates, E.A.; Jayes, K. But, who is the victim here? Exploring judgments toward hypothetical bidirectional domestic violence scenarios. *J. Interpers. Violence* **2022**, *37*, NP5495–NP5516. [CrossRef] [PubMed]
51. Capaldi, D.M.; Knoble, N.B.; Shortt, J.W.; Kim, H.K. A systematic review of risk factors for intimate partner violence. *Partn. Abus.* **2012**, *3*, 231–280. [CrossRef] [PubMed]
52. Abramsky, T.; Watts, C.H.; Garcia-Moreno, C.; Devries, K.; Kiss, L.; Ellsberg, M.; Jansen, H.A.; Heise, L. What factors are associated with recent intimate partner violence? Findings from the WHO multi-country study on women's health and domestic violence. *BMC Public Health* **2011**, *11*, 109. [CrossRef] [PubMed]
53. Rollero, C.; De Piccoli, N. Myths about Intimate Partner Violence and Moral Disengagement: An Analysis of Sociocultural Dimensions Sustaining Violence against Women. *Int. J. Environ. Res. Public Health* **2020**, *17*, 8139. [CrossRef]
54. García, V.; Lana, A.; Fernández, A.; Bringas, C.; Rodríguez-Franco, L.; Rodríguez-Díaz, J.J. Sexist attitudes and recognition of abuse in young couples. *Aten. Primaria* **2018**, *50*, 398–405.
55. Grabe, S. Promoting Gender Equality: The Role of Ideology, Power, and Control in the Link Between Land Ownership and Violence in Nicaragua. *Anal. Social. Issues Public Policy* **2010**, *10*, 146–170. [CrossRef]

56. Fine, S.L.; Kane, J.C.; Murray, S.M.; Skavenski, S.; Munthali, S.; Mwenge, M.; Paul, R.; Mayeya, J.; Murray, L.K. The role of violence acceptance and inequitable gender norms in intimate partner violence severity among couples in Zambia. *J. Interpers. Violence* **2021**, *36*, NP10744–NP10765. [CrossRef] [PubMed]
57. Wilchek-Aviad, Y.; Neeman-Haviv, V.; Shagan, N.; Ota-shushan, A. The public perception of female and male violence in marital relationships. *Smith Coll. Stud. Soc. Work* **2018**, *88*, 312–328. [CrossRef]
58. Yoshikawa, K.; Shakya, T.M.; Poudel, K.C.; Jimba, M. Agreement on reporting intimate partner violence among Nepalese couples: A cross-sectional study. *J. Interpers. Violence* **2018**, *886*, 312–328. [CrossRef]
59. Saldivar, A.; Díaz-Loving, R.; Reyes, N.; Armenta, C.; López, F.; Moreno, M.; Remero, A.; Hernández, J.; Domínguez, M. Roles de Género y Diversidad: Validación de una Escala en Varios Contextos Culturales. *Acta Investig. Psicológica* **2015**, *5*, 2124–2147.
60. Glick, P.; Fiske, S. The Ambivalence Toward Men Inventory. *Psychol. Women Q.* **1999**, *23*, 519–536. [CrossRef]
61. Carrión Briceño, M.L. Relaciones Entre La Ideología Política, El Sexismo Ambivalente y Los Estereotipos de Masculinidad Tradicional. Available online: https://tesis.pucp.edu.pe/repositorio/handle/20.500.12404/9933 (accessed on 3 March 2023).
62. Glick, P.; Fiske, S.T. Ambivalent sexism. *Adv. Exp. Soc. Psychol.* **2001**, *33*, 115–188. [CrossRef]
63. Bussey, K.; Fitzpatrick, S.; Raman, A. The role of moral disengagement and self-efficacy in cyberbullying. *J. Sch. Violence* **2015**, *14*, 30–46. [CrossRef]
64. Wang, X.; Yang, L.; Gao, L.; Yang, J.; Lei, L.; Wang, C. Childhood maltreatment and Chinese adolescents' bullying and defending: The mediating role of moral disengagement. *Child Abus. Negl.* **2017**, *69*, 134–144. [CrossRef]
65. Lamb, S.; Peterson, Z.D. Adolescent girls' sexual empowerment: Two feminists explore the concept. *Sex Roles* **2012**, *66*, 703–712. [CrossRef]
66. Lerum, K.; Dworkin, S.L. "Bad girls rule": An interdisciplinary feminist commentary on the report of the APA task force on the sexualization of girls. *J. Sex. Res.* **2009**, *46*, 250–263. [CrossRef]
67. Cuadrado Gordillo, I.; Fernández Antelo, I.; Martín-Mora Parra, G. ¿Pueden las víctimas de bullying convertirse en agresores del ciberespacio?: Estudio en población adolescente. *EJIHPE Eur. J. Investig. Health Psychol. Educ.* **2019**, *9*, 71–81. [CrossRef]
68. Olweus, D. Cyberbullying: An overrated phenomenon? *Eur. J. Dev. Psychol.* **2012**, *9*, 520–538. [CrossRef]
69. Del Rey, R.; Elipe, P.; Ortega-Ruiz, R. Bullying and cyberbullying: Overlapping and predictive value of the co-occurrence. *Psicothema* **2012**, *24*, 608–613.
70. Varjas, K.; Talley, J.; Meyers, J.; Parris, L.; Cutts, H. High school students' perceptions of motivations for cyberbullying: An exploratory study. *West J. Emerg. Med.* **2010**, *11*, 269.
71. Fleming, P.J.; Barrington, C.; Maman, S.; Lerebours, L.; Donastorg, Y.; Brito, M.O. Competition and humiliation: How masculine norms shape men's sexual and violent behaviors. *Men. Masc.* **2019**, *22*, 197–215. [CrossRef] [PubMed]
72. Vandello, J.A.; Bosson, J.K.; Cohen, D.; Burnaford, R.M.; Weaver, J.R. Precarious manhood. *J. Pers. Soc. Psychol.* **2008**, *95*, 1325. [CrossRef] [PubMed]
73. Vandello Joseph, A.; Bosson Jennifer, K. Hard won and easily lost: A review and synthesis of theory and research on precarious manhood. *Psychol. Men. Masc.* **2012**, *14*, 101–113. [CrossRef]
74. Cohen, D.; Nisbett, R.E. Self-protection and the culture of honor: Explaining southern violence. *Pers. Soc. Psychol. Bull.* **1994**, *20*, 551–567. [CrossRef]
75. Cohen, D.; Nisbett, R.E. Field experiments examining the culture of honor: The role of institutions in perpetuating norms about violence. *Pers. Soc. Psychol. Bull.* **1997**, *23*, 1188–1199. [CrossRef]

Disclaimer/Publisher's Note: The statements, opinions and data contained in all publications are solely those of the individual author(s) and contributor(s) and not of MDPI and/or the editor(s). MDPI and/or the editor(s) disclaim responsibility for any injury to people or property resulting from any ideas, methods, instructions or products referred to in the content.

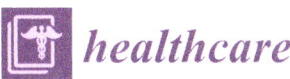

Review

The Risk Factors of Chronic Pain in Victims of Violence: A Scoping Review

Allison Uvelli [1,*], Cristina Duranti [1], Giulia Salvo [1], Anna Coluccia [1], Giacomo Gualtieri [2] and Fabio Ferretti [1]

1. Department of Medical Science, Surgery, and Neurosciences, University of Siena, Viale Bracci, 53100 Siena, Italy
2. Azienda Ospedaliero-Universitaria Senese (AOUS), Viale Bracci, 53100 Siena, Italy
* Correspondence: allison.uvelli@unisi.it; Tel.: +39-057-723-2517

Abstract: Violent situations are unfortunately very frequent in women and children all over the world. These experiences have long-term consequences for adult physical and psychological health. One of the most reported is chronic pain, defined in various sub-diagnoses and present in all types of violence. Unfortunately, the etiology of this condition is not clear and neither are the predisposing factors. The aim of this scoping review is to examine the literature trends about the probable risk factors of chronic pain in violence victims. Considering a bio-psycho-social model, it is possible to hypothesize the presence of all these aspects. The results will be discussed in the present article.

Keywords: risk factors; victims of violence; chronic pain; health; scoping review

1. Introduction

Childhood abuse and intimate partner violence (IPV) are two major global public health problems with serious adverse health consequences across life [1–3]. Every year, about 4–16% of children are physically abused and one in ten is neglected or psychologically abused [4]. Sexual abuse is experienced by 15–30% of girls and 5–15% of boys [4], and IPV is experienced by 35% of women [5]. The abuse involves all types of violence: sexual, physical, and psychological. Child maltreatment is more likely to occur in families afflicted with domestic violence and is associated with re-victimization in adulthood [6,7].

Evidence suggests that these experiences have long-term consequences on adult physical and psychological health [8,9]. The primary outcome is the onset of chronic pain [10], understood as the type of pain or discomfort in the involved area that tends to persist for at least 3 of the past 6 months. It is reported by 48% [11] to 84% [12] of abused women. The most common diagnosis of victimized are pelvic pain [13], fibromyalgia [14], irritable bowel syndrome/bowel symptoms [15], abdominal pain [16], migraine/headache [17], back pain [18], chest pain [19], and neck pain [20], which tend to become chronic as well as the pain derived from them. Unfortunately, the etiology of these conditions is not clear.

Previous studies found a relationship between chronic pain and specific psychological aspects [21], and neuroimaging studies showed that the activated brain areas by nociceptive stimuli are the same ones involved in emotional and behavioral states [22]. According to Garcia-Larrea and Peyron [23], pain elaboration involves three levels of neural connections. The first level processes the nociceptive activation of the spinothalamic tract. In the second level, the nociceptive stimulus is processed by the anterior cingulate cortex (ACC), insula, prefrontal cortex (PFC), and posterior parietal cortex, thanks to which the stimulus is consciously perceived, cognitively and attentionally modulated, and transformed into somatic or vegetative responses. The reappraisal of the stimulus takes place through the emotional context and individualized psychological factors that influence memory formation. The third level includes the orbitofrontal, perigenual ACC, and anterolateral PFC regions that can lead to inhibition or increase in the nociceptive stimulus perceived.

Citation: Uvelli, A.; Duranti, C.; Salvo, G.; Coluccia, A.; Gualtieri, G.; Ferretti, F. The Risk Factors of Chronic Pain in Victims of Violence: A Scoping Review. *Healthcare* **2023**, *11*, 2421. https://doi.org/10.3390/healthcare11172421

Academic Editors: Isabel Cuadrado-Gordillo and Parra Guadalupe Martín-Mora

Received: 18 July 2023
Revised: 1 August 2023
Accepted: 3 August 2023
Published: 29 August 2023

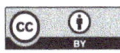

Copyright: © 2023 by the authors. Licensee MDPI, Basel, Switzerland. This article is an open access article distributed under the terms and conditions of the Creative Commons Attribution (CC BY) license (https://creativecommons.org/licenses/by/4.0/).

Mood disorders (depressive disorder, dysthymia, and bipolar disorder) are often present in chronic pain patients, ranging from 1% to 61% [24–26]. People affected by chronic pain were 2.0 to 2.5 times more likely to experience an episode of depression at 6- and 12-month follow-ups than individuals without chronic pain [27,28], and pain-free individuals with depressive disorder were 4 times more likely to develop chronic pain at 6- and 12 months follow-ups than not depressed individuals [29,30]. The cause–effect relationship would appear to be complicated and bidirectional. The same results were obtained for all anxiety disorders, whereas the prevalence in chronic pain patients ranged from 1% to 50%, with the same bidirectional relationship [31–33]. Also, for alcohol, drugs, and smoking, there is the same effect, with a prevalence of 1% to 25% [34–36]. Furthermore, suicidal thoughts are present in 28–48% of the cases [37,38], and violence doubles the odds of chronic pain onset [10].

Chronic pain, as opposed to acute pain, would seem to have little to do with injuries, even if it is still associated with biological processes; in fact, an interaction of sensory, autonomic, endocrine, and immune responses contribute to the nociceptive stimuli perceived [39]. The nervous system plays a role by detecting threats, signaling dangers, and starting a response to them, the endocrine system causes an arousal response to increase the survival odds thanks to the stress response, and the immune system detects microbial invasion and toxins and initiates complex inflammatory responses [40]. These processes could collectively compromise a defensive biological response to pain. Pain can persist as a focus of chronically disorganized, locally inflamed processes that respond maladaptively to systemic changes at the nervous, endocrine, and immune levels. In many chronic cases, the local tissue environment appears to repair itself, but sensory processes remain abnormal, creating chronic pain [39]. Trauma, such as violence and abuse, can cause the same biological reactions to nociceptive stimuli, activating the autonomic nervous system, which triggers the immune system and inflammatory response [41]. Inflammation can increase the risk of psychopathology by altering the metabolism of neurotransmitters, and psychopathology can similarly increase the risk of chronic pain [42].

Considering the complexity of the examined situation, the bio-psycho-social model [43] could help us to understand the phenomenon better. According to this model, the disease results from multiple variables: biological, psychological, and social, that co-occur in different ways for each person. Therefore, considering this approach, we might expect that the chronic pain in violence victims is not attributed exclusively to a single cause, psychological, sociological, or biological, but to a combination of the three. It remains to be understood in which way and prevalence these three categories are present in abused women.

This scoping review aims to analyze the research trends about the bio-psycho-social components most associated with chronic pain in victims of violence, considering all abuse types and the primary chronic pain diagnoses in violence cases. It is crucial to know them because if patients showed the major risk factors, preventive measures could be taken to counter the onset and/or chronicity of pain. This type of review does not exist in the literature, and thanks to it, it will be possible to increase the knowledge about this condition and help the victims from a clinical and research point of view. It would be possible to offer new solutions and therapeutic strategies from a clinical point of view and to orient studies about the creation of a new tool to evaluate the presence of these aspects.

2. Materials and Methods

This search protocol was based on the Preferred Reporting Items for Systematic Reviews and Meta-Analysis extension for Scoping Reviews (PRISMA-ScR) guidelines [44], according to the PECOS (Population, Exposure, Comparison, Outcome, Study Design) guidelines.

2.1. Search Strategy

The research was conducted on the electronic databases of PubMed, Scopus, Web of Science, and ERIC from March 2023 to June 2023 and we carried out a manual review of references. The search strategy relating to the risk factors of chronic pain in victims of violence was ("risk factor") AND ((pain)) AND ((("interpersonal violence" OR "domestic abuse" OR "intimate partner violence" OR "partner abuse" OR "violence against women"))). The keywords have been chosen after a preliminary search of the literature, thanks to which it was possible to identify the most used and relevant terms. There were no period restrictions on the search to increase the studies' yield, though the language was restricted to studies published in English or Italian. Authors were also contacted via email where there was insufficient data, and references from included studies were manually scanned for further sources as per published recommendations [45–47].

2.2. Criteria for Selection of Studies

It included studies on humans of any age with and without a history of abuse during their life identified through published observational study designs (cohort, case–control, and cross-sectional studies). An inclusive approach was adopted for the definition of abuse with a composite of sexual, physical, and psychological violence. Definitions of chronic pain varied between studies and it also adopted an inclusive approach. In general, whatever the type of pain or discomfort, it tends to persist in the involved area for at least 3 of the past 6 months. All bio-psycho-social risk factors were considered. Exclusion criteria included studies without a control group, studies without risk factors, and studies published in non-English or Italian languages. Lastly, systematic reviews, meta-analyses, commentaries, dissertations, thesis, editorials, and conference deeds were excluded but their references were examined to find other studies not retrieved by the search strategy.

2.3. Study Selection and Data Extraction

Studies were selected in a three-stage process. All citations identified from initial searching were imported into Zotero Software, where duplicate citations were removed, and after which, two reviewers (AU & CD) independently scrutinized all article titles remaining from the original search. After this, the same two reviewers independently analyzed all article abstracts remaining from the second removal. If there was a disagreement, an independent third reviewer (FF) was consulted. If the abstracts did not provide sufficient information to determine inclusion or exclusion, the reference was included in the next stage (full-text screening) to confirm the information in the full text. Full manuscripts were obtained for studies meeting initial inclusion criteria, and two reviewers (AU & GS) carried out an independent full-text review of all English/Italian language articles. The most recent and complete version of duplicate publications was included in the full-text review, and inadequate versions were excluded. Disagreements regarding inclusion or exclusion criteria were resolved by consensus or consultation of an independent third reviewer (FF). Two reviewers (AU & CD) performed independent data extraction, and where extractable data were missing, authors were contacted by email. They used data to construct tables of risk factors.

2.4. Assessment of Study Quality

All studies meeting the selection criteria were assessed for quality based on existing checklists [48]. Quality was defined as the confidence that bias in estimating the effect of risk factors on pain symptom outcomes in victims of violence was minimized through appropriate study design methods and analysis. Two reviewers (AU & GS) independently assessed all studies for quality using predetermined and validated criteria from The Johanna Briggs Institute appraisal checklists for cross-sectional, case–control, and cohort studies [48]. Appraisal criteria included comparability and appropriateness of cases and controls, reliable and valid exposure measurement, identification of confounding factors and whether strategies were implemented to deal with these factors, valid and reliable outcomes assessment, and appropriateness of statistical analyses used. A high-quality study was considered to meet most of these criteria: cross-sectional studies met at least 5/8 criteria, cohort studies fulfilled at least 6/11, and case–control studies met at least 6/10. Low-quality studies were excluded from our review. Cohort studies satisfy

7/11 criteria, 2 case–control studies satisfy 7/10, 2 of them 8/10, 6 cross-sectional studies satisfy 5/8 criteria, 3 satisfy 7/8 criteria, and the last 10 satisfy 6/8 criteria. The utilized appraisal checklists are available as Supplementary Materials.

3. Results

3.1. Literature Identification, Study Characteristics, and Quality

The search protocol identified 116 publications from online databases. There were 17 removed as they were duplicate publications. The remaining 99 studies were screened against title and abstract criteria, after which 51 were excluded. Of the 48 studies selected for full-text review, 23 were excluded, 3 were reviews, 6 were written in unknown languages, 5 had no pain condition, 5 had pain caused by an injury, and 4 focused on the offender's group. After, the quality assessment was carried out on 25 studies [49–73]; see the flow diagram in Figure 1.

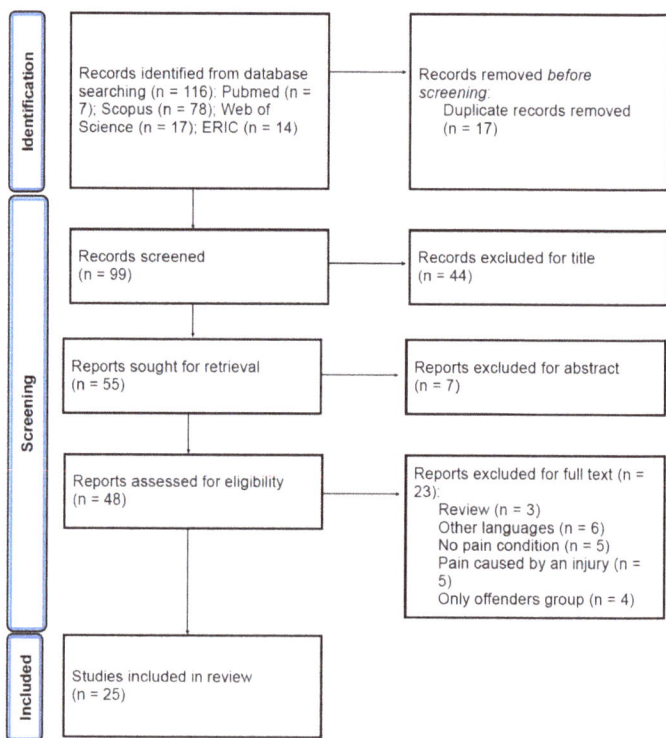

Figure 1. PRISMA flowchart [74].

The years of the studies range from 2004 to 2022; 19 studies are cross-sectional, 4 are case–control, and 2 are cohort studies. Of the included studies, 44% are from the United States of America (USA) (11), 12% are from Australia (3), 8% are from Canada (2), and 36% are from other countries (Spain, Thailand, Brazil, Slovenia, Turkey, Serbia, Pakistan, Oman, South Africa). The sample size ranges from 23,846 to 37, age ranges from 15 to 98, and all the abuse and chronic pain types are represented.

3.2. Risk Factors

According to the bio-psycho-social model [43] and what was found in the selected studies, there are three specific categories of risk factors: biological, psychological, and sociological. Of these categories, the biological one can be divided into weight conditions, acute upper/lower respiratory tract affection, genitourinary conditions, cardiovascular symptoms and conditions, endocrine disease, hormonal conditions, gastrointestinal disorders, skin problems, and specific inflammations. The psycho-social risk factors can be divided into mental health disease, use of psychoactive substances, life events, life quality, and personal characteristics. Inside the 14 categories, there are many signs, symptoms, and conditions, for a total of 65, as described in Table 1.

Table 1. List of risk factors divided into categories.

Biological Risk Factors	Psycho-Social Risk Factors
Weight condition <ul><li>Obesity</li><li>Underweight</li></ul> **Acute upper/lower respiratory tract affection** <ul><li>Asthma</li><li>Allergic rhinitis</li><li>Sinusitis</li><li>Nasal congestion</li></ul> **Genitourinary conditions** <ul><li>Sexually transmitted infections (AIDS, chlamydia)</li><li>Genital infections (vaginitis, vulvitis, cervicitis)</li><li>Urinary tract infections (cystitis, urethritis)</li><li>Vaginal bulge</li><li>Urinary leakage</li><li>Genital vesicles/ulcers</li><li>Postcoital bleeding</li><li>Prolapse</li></ul> **Cardiovascular symptoms and conditions** <ul><li>Hypertension</li><li>Heart palpitation</li></ul> **Endocrine disease** <ul><li>Disorder of lipid metabolism</li><li>Diabetes</li><li>Thyroid disease</li><li>High cholesterol</li></ul> **Hormonal conditions** <ul><li>Menopausal symptoms</li><li>Dysmenorrhea/irregular menstrual cycle</li></ul> **Gastrointestinal disorders** <ul><li>Gastroesophageal reflux</li><li>Irregularities in bowel functioning (diarrohea, constipation, dischezia)</li></ul> **Skin problems** <ul><li>Dermatitis</li><li>Eczema</li><li>Rash</li></ul> **Specific inflammations** <ul><li>Otitis</li><li>Conjunctivitis</li><li>Muscle inflammation</li><li>Osteoarthritis</li></ul>	**Mental health disease** <ul><li>Sleeping disorders</li><li>Anxiety disorders</li><li>Depressive disorders</li><li>Mood disorders</li><li>Post-traumatic stress disorder (PTSD)</li><li>Psychosomatic disorders</li><li>Eating disorders</li><li>History of psychiatric disorders</li></ul> **Use of psychoactive substances** <ul><li>Drugs</li><li>Alcohol</li><li>Smoking</li></ul> **Life events** <ul><li>Intimate partner violence (IPV)</li><li>Childhood abuse</li><li>Witnessing violence (including in ACEs)</li><li>Adverse childhood experiences (ACEs)</li><li>Parental psychopathology</li><li>Parental marital conflict</li><li>Poor parent–child relationship</li><li>Number of abuse (revictimization)</li><li>Abortion</li></ul> **Life quality** <ul><li>Life dissatisfaction</li><li>Mental distress</li><li>Suicidal thoughts</li><li>Feeling of shame and guilty</li><li>Low self-esteem</li><li>Sexual dissatisfaction</li><li>Family and social problem</li><li>Low social support</li><li>Reduced physical functioning/physical inactivity</li></ul> **Personal characteristics** <ul><li>Role emotional</li><li>Tiredness</li><li>Low vitality</li><li>Number of sexual partner</li><li>Age of first sexual intercourse/sex too soon</li><li>Painful intercourse</li></ul>

3.3. The Impact of Risk Factors in the Studies

The selected studies give information about the complexity of the treated problem; in fact, each of them includes both biological and psycho-social aspects. All 25 studies involve psycho-social conditions, and 14 also involve biological conditions.

3.3.1. Biological Risk Factors

Within the biological risk factors, weight conditions are present in 20% of the studies; five are about obesity, and one is about an underweight condition. Acute upper/lower respiratory tract affections are present in 12% of the studies; in three, the specific conditions are asthma, allergic rhinitis, and sinusitis, and in one, it is nasal congestion. Genitourinary conditions are reported in 40% of the studies; in five of them, there are urinary tract infections, in three of them, there are sexually transmitted infections and genital infections, and in one case, there is a vaginal bulge, urinary leakage, genital vesicles, genital ulcers, postcoital bleeding, or prolapse. Cardiovascular symptoms and conditions are reported in 24% of the studies; in five, the condition is hypertension, and in one, it is heart palpitation. Endocrine diseases are present in 12% of the studies; in three, there is diabetes, and in one, there is a disorder of lipid metabolism, thyroid disease, or high cholesterol. In 8% of the studies, they reported a hormonal condition that involved menopausal symptoms one time and dysmenorrhea/irregular menstrual cycle two times. In 20% of the studies, they reported a gastrointestinal disorder that involved irregularities in bowel functioning four times and gastroesophageal reflux one time. Skin problems are present in 8% of the studies; in one, there is dermatitis and eczema, and in the other, there is a rash. Lastly, specific inflammations are reported in 12% of the studies; one time regarding otitis and conjunctivitis, one time regarding muscle inflammation, and one time regarding osteoarthritis.

3.3.2. Psycho-Social Risk Factors

Inside the psycho-social risk factors, mental health diseases are present in 64% of the studies; 13 of them involved a depressive or mood disorder, 9 of them an anxiety disorder, 6 of them a sleep disorder, 4 of them PTSD, 3 a psychosomatic disorder, and in one case, an eating disorder or general history of psychiatric disorder. The use of psychoactive substances is reported in 36% of the studies, presenting drugs and alcohol use in five cases, respectively, and smoking in six cases. Specific life events are noticed in 100% of the studies; in particular, are always-present IPV referred to in 18 studies, childhood abuse, referred to in 3 studies, and both, referred to in 4 studies. Following this, ACEs and parental psychopathology are referred to in two studies, respectively, and parental marital conflict, poor parent–child relationship, abortions, and re-victimization are referred to in one study, respectively. In 24% of the studies, they referred to a life quality condition; in two cases, it concerned life dissatisfaction, mental distress, and suicidal thoughts, and in one case, it concerns feelings of shame and guilt, low self-esteem, sexual dissatisfaction, family/social problems, low social support, reduced physical functioning/physical inactivity. Lastly, 24% of the studies refer to at least one of the following characteristics: role of emotions, tiredness, low vitality, and number of sexual partners in one case, the age of first sexual intercourse/sex too soon in two cases, and painful intercourse in four cases. These results are summarized in Table 2.

Table 2. Characteristics and results of the included studies.

Authors	Sample	Study Design	Pain	Risk Factors
Ali et al. (2021) Pakistan [69]	945 F 15–49 y/o	Cross-sectional	Pelvic pain	• Life events (1): IPV • Personal (1): painful intercourse • Hormonal (1): dysmenorrhea • Genitourinary (7): urinary tract infections, genital infections, urinary leakage, genital vescicles/ulcers, postcoital bleeding, and prolapse
Al Kendi et al. (2021) Oman [70]	978 F 30.6 y/o	Cross-sectional	General chronic pain	• Life events (1): IPV • Mental health (3): depression, sleeping, and psychosomatic disorders
Bonomi et al. (2007) USA [50]	1928 F 18–64 y/o	Cross-sectional	General chronic pain	• Life events (1): IPV • Life quality (1): family and social problems • Mental health (3): sleeping, anxiety, and depressive disorders • Substances (2): smoking and drugs • Respiratory (3): allergic rhinitis, asthma, and sinusitis • Cardiovascular (1): hypertension • Endocrine (3): disorder of lipid metabolism, thyroid disease, and diabetes • Inflammations (2): otitis and conjunctivitis • Genitourinary (2): genital infections and urinary tract infections • Hormonal (2): menopausal symptoms and irregular menstrual cycle • Gastrointestinal (1): gastroesophageal reflux • Skin (2): dermatitis and eczema • Weight: obesity
Chartier et al. (2010) Canada [52]	9953 (5187 F—4766 M) 15–98 y/o	Cross-sectional	General chronic pain	• Life events (4): childhood abuse, parental marital conflict, parental psychopathology, and poor parent–child relationship
De Wet-Billings & Godongwana (2021) South Africa [71]	216 F 15–34 y/o	Cross-sectional	General chronic pain	• Life events (2): IPV • Cardiovascular (1): hypertension
England-Mason et al. (2018) Canada [64]	23,846 (12,290 F—11,556 M) 18–64 y/o	Cross-sectional	General chronic pain	• Life events (2): childhood abuse and witnessing violence • Mental health (2): mood and anxiety disorders • Substances (2): smoking and drugs
Eslick et al. (2011) Australia [55]	87 (66 F—21 M) 47 y/o	Case-control	General chronic pain	• Life events (1): childhood abuse • Mental health (1): depressive disorder

21

Table 2. *Cont.*

Authors	Sample	Study Design	Pain	Risk Factors
FitzPatrick et al. (2022) Australia [72]	1507 F 31 y/o	Cohort	Pelvic pain	• Life events (1): IPV • Mental health (2): anxiety and depression disorders • Personal (2): age of first sexual intercourse and painful intercourse • Genitourinary (1): urinary leakage • Weight: obesity
Gelaye et al. (2016) USA [61]	2970 F 28.1 y/o	Cross-sectional	General chronic pain	• Life events (3): IPV, childhood abuse, and number of abuse
Gerber et al. (2017) USA [58]	92 F 39 y/o	Cross-sectional	General chronic pain	• Life events (1): IPV • Mental health (1): PTSD • Substances (2): smoking and alcohol
Grossi et al. (2018) Brazil [65]	80 F 33 y/o	Case-control	General chronic pain	• Life events (1): IPV • Mental health (2): depression and psychosomatic disorders
Gucek & Selic (2018) Slovenia [66]	161 F 51.1 y/o	Cross-sectional	General chronic pain	• Life events (1): IPV • Mental health (5): depression, anxiety, sleeping, eating, and psychosomatic disorders • Life quality (3): reduced physical functioning, feelings of shame and guilty, and low self-esteem • Substances (1): smoking • Inflammations (1): muscle • Gastrointestinal (1): irregularities in bowel functioning • Genitourinary (2): genital infections and urinary tract infections
Gunduz et al. (2019) Turkey [67]	136 F 40 y/o	Case-control	Fibromyalgia	• Life events (2): IPV and parental psychopathology • Mental health (4): history of psychiatric disorder, PTSD, mood, and anxiety disorders • Substances (2): smoking and alcohol
Halpern et al. (2017) USA [62]	37 F 19-63 y/o	Cross-sectional	General chronic pain	• Life events (1): IPV • Mental health (2): PTSD and anxiety disorder • Cardiovascular (2): heart palpitation, hypertension

Table 2. Cont.

Authors	Sample	Study Design	Pain	Risk Factors
Hegarty et al. (2008) Australia [51]	942 F 16–50 y/o	Cross-sectional	General chronic pain	• Life events (1): IPV • Mental health (3): depression, anxiety, and sleeping disorders • Personal (1): tiredness • Life quality (1): suicidal thoughts • Genitourinary (1): urinary leakage • Gastrointestinal (1): irregularities in bowel functioning • Respiratory (1): nasal congestion • Skin (1): rash • Cardiovascular (1): hypertension
Jovanovic et al. (2020) Serbia [68]	6320 F 20–75 y/o	Cross-sectional	General chronic pain	• Life events (2): IPV and abortions • Mental health (2): depression and sleeping disorders • Substances (1): alcohol
Kelly et al. (2011) USA [56]	135 F 40.3 y/o	Cross-sectional	General chronic pain	• Life events (2): childhood abuse and IPV • Mental health (4): PTSD, sleeping, depression, and anxiety disorders • Life quality (2): life dissatisfaction and suicidal thoughts
Lutgendorf et al. (2017) USA [63]	188 F 18–64 y/o	Cross-sectional	Pelvic pain	• Life events (1): IPV • Personal (1): painful intercourse • Genitourinary (1): vaginal bulge • Gastrointestinal (1): irregularities in bowel functioning
Parish et al. (2004) USA [49]	3323 (1662 F—1661 M) 20–64 y/o	Cross-sectional	General chronic pain	• Life events (1): IPV • Life quality (3): life, mental, and sexual dissatisfaction • Genitourinary (1): sexually transmitted infections
Raphael et al. (2022) USA [73]	1974 F 60.2 y/o	Cross-sectional	Pelvic pain	• Life events (1): IPV • Mental health (1): depression disorders • Genitourinary (1): urinary tract infections • Endocrine (1): diabetes • Weight: obesity and underweight
Saito et al. (2013) Thailand [59]	421 F 25.9 y/o	Cross-sectional	General chronic pain	• Life events (1): IPV • Personal (2): role emotional and low vitality • Mental health (1): depressive disorder

Table 2. Cont.

Authors	Sample	Study Design	Pain	Risk Factors
Sutherland et al. (2013) USA [60]	145 F 30.1 y/o	Cross-sectional	Pelvic pain	• Life events (2): IPV and childhood abuse • Personal (3): number of sexual partner, painful intercourse, and age of first sexual intercourse • Substances (2): alcohol and drugs • Genitourinary (2): sexually transmitted infections and urinary tract infections
Vives-Cases et al. (2010) Spain [53]	13,094 F 16–64 y/o	Cross-sectional	General chronic pain	• Life events (1): IPV • Life quality (2): low social support and mental distress • Substances (2): smoking and drugs • Cardiovascular (1): hypertension • Weight: obesity
Williams et al. (2010) USA [54]	309 F 18–64 y/o	Case-control	Pelvic pain	• Life events (2): childhood abuse and IPV • Genitourinary (1): sexually transmitted infections
Young et al. (2011) USA [57]	360 (260 F—100 M) 53 y/o	Cohort	General chronic pain	• Life events (2): IPV and ACEs • Mental health (2): depression and anxiety disorders • Substances (2): alcohol and drugs • Inflammations (1): osteoarthritis • Respiratory (1): asthma • Endocrine (2): diabetes and high cholesterol • Gastrointestinal (1): irregularities in bowel functioning • Cardiovascular (2): hypertension and hearth palpitation • Weight: obesity

4. Discussion

This study aimed to explore the bio-psycho-social factors strongly correlated to the onset of chronic pain in violence victims. Therefore, a scoping review was conducted, and now it is possible to make some considerations.

4.1. The Most Common Conditions

This scoping review showed a significant trend for the psycho-social aspects of the phenomenon. They are present in all the included studies and have the central frequency inside the categories. Considering 14 categories, of which 9 are biological, and 5 are psycho-social, and life events and mental health diseases have a prevalence of 25% and 16%, respectively, the most significant two. In particular, the abuse conditions (IPV and childhood abuse), adverse experiences, and mood, depressive and anxiety disorders (PTSD included) are the most reported. This evidence is in line with studies that showed a relationship between violence and chronic pain [9,10], and some mental health diagnoses and chronic pain [24–33]. A particular condition is related to sleeping disorders. There is a literature trend of their involvement, but previous studies do not report a clear and direct relationship with chronic pain or violence. Also in the included studies, they are always present with depression and anxiety disorders comorbidity and never individually. They could be referred to as a secondary diagnosis or a symptom of other conditions, rather than a diagnosis in itself. The nonspecific psychopathology, eating, and psychosomatic disorders would appear less frequent, such as parental marital conflict, poor parent–child relationship, parental psychopathology, and re-victimization. Also, in these cases, the relationship may not be direct but instead increases the odds of the onset of another clinical condition, increasing the odds of the onset of chronic pain.

The genitourinary conditions category has a prevalence of 10%, with a significant trend in urinary tract, genital, and sexually transmitted infections. These could be caused by sexual violence, inducing chronic pelvic pain [75]. Unfortunately, this association is not only for sexually abused but also for the other types. In this case, it is possible to hypothesize a concomitance of biological and psychological aspects involving life quality and personal characteristics components. On the one hand, there are biological infections; on the other hand, maybe there is sexual dissatisfaction, having first sexual intercourse at an age in which there are not adequate cognitive abilities to process the experience, and painful intercourse, which can be both infectious and traumatic. Vaginal bulge, urinary leakage, genital vesicles/ulcers, postcoital bleeding, and prolapse are minor influences in determining chronic pain and can be symptoms or not of the primary diagnoses. In personal characteristics, which have a prevalence of 6%, the only two influential elements are those related to sexual/genital/urinary infections: sex too soon and painful intercourse. The number of sexual partners, emotions, tiredness, and low vitality are not. Tiredness and low vitality may be present later due to chronic pain rather than as an underlying vulnerability.

The use of psychoactive substances has a trend of 9% and is in line with studies that showed a bidirectional relationship with chronic pain [34–36]. Their use could interfere with the neural process of restoration of homeostatic conditions and then be used to manage pain.

Life quality and cardiovascular symptoms and conditions have a trend of 6%, with life dissatisfaction, mental distress, suicidal thoughts, hypertension, and heart palpitation as the most referred to. There could be a link between mental distress and cardiovascular conditions; in fact, hypertension and heart palpitations are both influenced by high stress levels [76,77]. Violence causes increased stress [78], which causes hypertension and heart palpitations that predispose to chronic chest pain [19]. Also, suicidal thoughts are influenced by stress [79], and their prevalence is in line with studies that showed a bidirectional relationship with chronic pain [37,38]. Feelings of shame and guilt, low self-esteem, family and social problems, low social support, and physical inactivity are less critical in the life quality category. Low self-esteem is more of a risk factor for IPV than chronic pain in victims [80], and family/social problems and low social support, and feelings of shame and guilt are those referred to after the violence. Instead, physical inactivity is a consequence of pain.

4.2. Other Conditions

Weight conditions and gastrointestinal disorders have a trend of 5%; in particular, present are obesity and irregularities in bowel functioning, being less underweight, and gastroesophageal reflux. Clear evidence has shown a link between IPV and obesity [81,82], and PTSD and depression have a crucial mediating role in this [83,84]. The pathway through which the severity of abuse leads to obesity is similar to the mechanism by which obesity and chronic pain exacerbate each other [85]. For the specific irregularities in bowel functioning cases, the evidence is still unclear.

Acute upper/lower respiratory tract affection, endocrine diseases, and specific inflammations have a trend of 3%, and the most reported conditions are asthma and diabetes; allergic rhinitis, sinusitis, nasal congestion, disorder of lipid metabolism, thyroid disease, high cholesterol, and all of the specific inflammations appear to be indirectly related to chronic pain in violence victims. Previous studies found that several factors contribute to the risk of developing asthma, including obesity, female sex, high levels of family stress, and IPV [86–88], and experimental studies have yielded novel insight into the potential pathways underlying the connection between these conditions and chronic pain, such as stress-related changes in epigenetic processes, gene expression, and immune responses [89]. Adler [90] has already found a correlation between inflammations and chronic pain, and it is clear that the reason for its presence in this specific sample is probably that it is an a-specific risk factor.

Lastly, skin problems and hormonal conditions have a trend of 2%, with dysmenorrhea/irregular menstrual cycles as the most reported situation. Skin problems, such as dermatitis, eczema, and rash, are related to stress levels, which worsen them [91]. The brain areas related to chronic pain and some psychiatric conditions (e.g., dorsolateral PFC) could significantly influence the skin problem progression, but also, in this case, there is not a direct effect on IPV. John and colleagues [92] and Letourneau and colleagues [93] found an association between violence and dysmenorrhea/irregular menstrual cycles, in particular for sexual or physical violence [94], that increases the risk of the onset of pelvic pain [95], but the reasons of this association need further investigations.

4.3. Limitations

This study has some limitations: First, the research method is a scoping review. PRISMA-ScR and PECOS guidelines are used to fill this gap, and a quality assessment was conducted, but other sources of information are excluded, and the grey literature has not been sufficiently analyzed. Then, the non-English/Italian article exclusion leads to the non-inclusion of six potentially relevant articles. Moreover, the inclusion of only observational study designs, due to the absence of interventional studies, may make the results less generalizable. Furthermore, the included studies are not enough to totally clarify the research question. Future directions of this topic will have to increase the number of studies and then conduct a systematic review.

5. Conclusions

Intimate partner violence is a health problem that has many physical and psychological consequences, including chronic pain. This study showed that some biological and psycho-social components increase the odds of chronic pain onset. Unfortunately, how they interact with each other is not yet fully established. By continuing the studies in this direction, it will be possible exactly establish the specific and a-specific risk factors and their relationships. After that, it could be possible to create a screening tool to direct women to the correct treatment and individualized treatment that is not possible at the moment because the specific considerable variables were unknown. Surely, future studies could investigate the relationship between biological and psycho-social risk factors to establish cause–effect associations, and to understand which of those found in the trends are relevant in these patients. Despite the limitations, the presenting study is the first to examine the literature trends about factors that accompanied chronic pain in violence victims.

Supplementary Materials: The following supporting information can be downloaded at: https://www.mdpi.com/article/10.3390/healthcare11172421/s1, Summary of quality assessment.

Author Contributions: A.U., C.D. and G.S. have been involved in conceptualization, methodology, data extraction, and curation. F.F. has participated in data curation, analysis, and methodology. G.G. and A.C. have participated in conceptualization, and A.U. and F.F. in manuscript writing. All authors have read and agreed to the published version of the manuscript.

Funding: This APC was funded by the University of Siena, Department of Medical Science, Surgery and Neurosciences, Italy.

Institutional Review Board Statement: Not applicable.

Informed Consent Statement: Not applicable.

Data Availability Statement: The data reported here, and the quality assessment tables and checklists are available upon request.

Conflicts of Interest: The authors declare no conflict of interest.

References

1. Sachs-Ericsson, N.; Blazer, D.; Plant, E.A.; Arnow, B. Childhood sexual and physical abuse and the 1-year prevalence of medical problems in the National Comorbidity Survey. *Health Psychol.* **2005**, *24*, 32–40. [CrossRef] [PubMed]
2. Danese, A.; Moffitt, T.E.; Harrington, H.; Milne, B.J.; Polanczyk, G.; Pariante, C.M.; Poulton, R.; Caspi, A. Adverse childhood experiences and adult risk factors for age-related disease: Depression, inflammation, and clustering of metabolic risk markers. *Arch. Pediatr. Adolesc.* **2009**, *163*, 1135–1143. [CrossRef] [PubMed]
3. Garcia-Moreno, C.; Heise, L.; Jansen, H.A.; Ellsberg, M.; Watts, C. Public health. Violence against women. *Science* **2005**, *310*, 1282–1283. [CrossRef] [PubMed]
4. Gilbert, R.; Spatz Widom, C.; Browne, K.; Fergusson, D.; Webb, E.; Janson, S. Burden and consequences of child maltreatment in high-income countries. *Lancet* **2009**, *373*, 68–81. [CrossRef]
5. World Health Organization. World Report on Violence and Health. Available online: https://www.who.int/publications/i/item/9241545615 (accessed on 3 October 2022).
6. Graham-Bermann, S.A. Child abuse in the context of domestic violence. In *The APSAC Handbook on Child Maltreatment*; Myers, J.E.B., Berliner, L., Briere, J., Hendrix, C.T., Jenny, C., Reid, T.A., Eds.; Sage Publications: Thousand Oaks, CA, USA, 2002; Volume 1, pp. 119–130.
7. Kwon, M.; You, S. Gender and role associations between domestic violence during childhood and dating violence: Victimization among male college students mediated through violence justification beliefs. *Child. Abuse Negl.* **2023**, *141*, 106233. [CrossRef]
8. Cirici, A.R.; Soler, A.R.; Cobo, J.; Soldevilla, A.J.M. Psychological consequences and daily life adjustment for victims of intimate partner violence. *Int. J. Psychiatry Med.* **2023**, *58*, 6–19. [CrossRef]
9. Bussieres, A.; Hartvigsen, J.; Ferreira, M.L.; Ferreira, P.H.; Hancock, M.J.; Stone, L.S.; Wideman, T.H.; Boruff, J.; Elklit, A. Adverse childhood experience and adult persistent pain and disability: Protocol for a systematic review and meta-analysis. *Syst. Rev.* **2020**, *9*, 215. [CrossRef]
10. Uvelli, A.; Ribaudo, C.; Gualtieri, G.; Coluccia, A.; Ferretti, F. The association between violence against women and chronic pain: A systematic review and meta-analysis. *Res. Sq.* **2023**, *under review*. [CrossRef]
11. Campbell, J.C. Health consequences of intimate partner violence. *Lancet* **2002**, *359*, 1331–1336. [CrossRef]
12. Sutherland, C.A.; Bybee, D.I.; Sullivan, C.M. Beyond bruises and broken bones: The joint effects of stress and injuries on battered women's health. *Am. J. Community Psychol.* **2002**, *30*, 609–636. [CrossRef]
13. As-Sanie, S.; Clevenger, L.A.; Geisser, M.E.; Williams, D.A.; Roth, R.S. History of abuse and its relationship to pain experience and depression in women with chronic pelvic pain. *Am. J. Obstet. Gynecol.* **2014**, *210*, 317.e1–317.e8. [CrossRef]
14. Chandan, J.S.; Thomas, T.; Raza, K.; Bradbury-Jones, C.; Taylor, J.; Bandyopadhyay, S.; Nirantharakumar, K. Intimate partner violence and the risk of developing fibromyalgia and chronic fatigue syndrome. *J. Interpers. Violence* **2021**, *36*, NP12279–NP12298. [CrossRef] [PubMed]
15. Ringel, Y.; Whitehead, W.E.; Toner, B.B.; Diamant, N.E.; Hu, Y.; Jia, H.; Bangdiwala, S.I.; Drossman, D.A. Sexual and physical abuse are not associated with rectal hypersensitivity in patients with irritable bowel syndrome. *Gut* **2004**, *53*, 838–842. [CrossRef]
16. Bo, M.; Canavese, A.; Magnano, L.; Rondana, A.; Castagna, P.; Gino, S. Violence against pregnant women in the experience of the rape centre of Turin: Clinical and forensic evaluation. *J. Forensic Leg. Med.* **2020**, *76*, 102071. [CrossRef]

17. Cripe, S.M.; Sanchez, S.E.; Gelaye, B.; Sanchez, E.; Williams, M.A. Association between intimate partner violence, migraine, and probable migraine. *Headache* **2011**, *51*, 208–219. [CrossRef] [PubMed]
18. Wuest, J.; Merritt-Gray, M.; Ford-Gilboe, M.; Lent, B.; Varcoe, C.; Campbell, J.C. Chronic pain in women survivors of intimate partner violence. *J. Pain* **2008**, *9*, 1049–1057. [CrossRef] [PubMed]
19. Coll-Vinent, B.; Marti, G.; Calderon, S.; Martinez, B.; Cespedes, F.; Fuenzalida, C. La violencia de pareja en las pacientes que consultan pr dolor toracico en urgencias. *Semergen* **2018**, *45*, 23–29. [CrossRef]
20. Shields, L.B.; Corey, T.S.; Weakley-Jones, B.; Stewart, D. Living victims of strangulation: A 10-year review of cases in a metropolitan community. *Am. J. Forensic Med. Pathol.* **2010**, *31*, 320–325. [CrossRef]
21. .Melzack, R. Phantom limbs and the concept of a neuromatrix. *Trends Neurosci.* **1990**, *13*, 88–92. [CrossRef]
22. Baliki, M.N.; Apkarian, A.V. Nociception, pain, negative moods, and behavior selection. *Neuron* **2015**, *87*, 474–491. [CrossRef]
23. Garcia-Larrea, L.; Peyron, R. Pain matrices and neuropathic pain matrices: A review. *Pain* **2013**, *154*, S29–S43. [CrossRef]
24. Raphael, K.G.; Janal, M.N.; Nayak, S.; Schwartz, J.E.; Gallagher, R.M. Psychiatric comorbidities in a community sample of women with fibromyalgia. *Pain* **2006**, *124*, 117–125. [CrossRef] [PubMed]
25. Uguz, F.; Cicek, E.; Salli, A.; Karahan, A.Y.; Albayrak, I.; Kaya, N.; Ugurlu, H. Axis I and Axis II psychiatric disorders in patients with fibromyalgia. *Gen. Hosp. Psychiatry* **2010**, *32*, 105–107. [CrossRef] [PubMed]
26. Kudlow, P.A.; Rosenblat, J.D.; Weissman, C.R.; Cha, D.S.; Kakar, R.; McIntyre, R.S.; Sharma, V. Prevalence of fibromyalgia and co-morbid bipolar disorder: A systematic review and meta-analysis. *J. Affect. Disord.* **2015**, *188*, 134–142. [CrossRef] [PubMed]
27. Carroll, L.J.; Cassidy, J.D.; Cote, P. Factors associated with the onset of an episode of depressive symptoms in the general population. *J. Clin. Epidemiol.* **2003**, *56*, 651–658. [CrossRef] [PubMed]
28. Currie, S.R.; Wang, J. Chronic back pain and major depression in the general Canadian population. *Pain* **2004**, *107*, 54–60. [CrossRef] [PubMed]
29. Carroll, L.J.; Cassidy, J.D.; Cote, P. Depression as a risk factor for onset of an episode of troublesome neck and low back pain. *Pain* **2004**, *107*, 134–139. [CrossRef]
30. Currie, S.R.; Wang, J. More data on major depression as an antecedent risk factors for first onset of chronic back pain. *Psychol. Med.* **2005**, *35*, 1275–1282. [CrossRef]
31. Von Korff, M.; Crane, P.; Lane, M.; Miglioretti, D.L.; Simon, G.; Saunders, K.; Stang, P.; Brandenburg, N.; Kessler, R. Chronic spinal pain and physical-mental comorbidity in the United States: Results from the national comorbidity survey replication. *Pain* **2005**, *113*, 331–339. [CrossRef]
32. Stang, P.E.; Brandenburg, N.A.; Lane, M.C.; Merikangas, K.R.; Von Korff, M.R.; Kessler, R.C. Mental and physical comorbid conditions and days in role among persons with arthritis. *Psychosom. Med.* **2006**, *68*, 152–158. [CrossRef]
33. Demyttenaere, K.; Bruffaerts, R.; Lee, S.; Posada-Villa, J.; Kovess, V.; Angermeyer, M.C.; Levinson, D.; de Girolamo, G.; Nakane, H.; Mneimneh, Z.; et al. Mental disorders among persons with chronic back or neck pain: Results from the World Mental Health Survey. *Pain* **2007**, *129*, 332–342. [CrossRef]
34. Arnold, L.M.; Hudson, J.I.; Keck, P.E.; Auchenbach, M.B.; Javaras, K.N.; Hess, E.V. Comorbidity of fibromyalgia and psychiatric disorders. *J. Clin. Psychiatry* **2006**, *67*, 1219–1225. [CrossRef] [PubMed]
35. Zhao, Y.; Liu, J.; Zhao, Y.; Thethi, T.; Fonseca, V.; Shi, L. Predictors of duloxetine versus other treatments among veterans with diabetic peripheral neuropathic pain: A retrospective study. *Pain Pract.* **2012**, *12*, 366–373. [CrossRef] [PubMed]
36. Alonso-Moran, E.; Orueta, J.F.; Fraile Esteban, J.I.; Arteagoitia Axpe, J.M.; Marques Gonzalez, M.L.; Toro Polanco, N.; Ezkurra Loiola, P.; Gaztambide, S.; Nuno-Solinis, R. The prevalence of diabetes-related complications and multimorbidity in the population with type 2 diabetes mellitus in the Basque Country. *BMC Public Health* **2014**, *14*, 1059. [CrossRef] [PubMed]
37. Cheatle, M.D.; Wasser, T.; Foster, C.; Olugbodi, A.; Bryan, J. Prevalence of suicidal ideation in patients with chronic non-cancer pain referred to a behaviorally based pain program. *Pain Physician* **2014**, *17*, E359–E367. [CrossRef]
38. Trinanes, Y.; Gonzalez-Villar, A.; Gomez-Perretta, C.; Carrillo-de-la-Pena, M.T. Suicidality in chronic pain: Predictors of suicidal ideation in fibromyalgia. *Pain Pract.* **2015**, *15*, 323–332. [CrossRef] [PubMed]
39. Chapman, C.R.; Tuckett, R.P.; Woo Song, C. Pain and stress in systems perspective: Reciprocal neural, endocrine and immune interactions. *J. Pain* **2008**, *9*, 122–145. [CrossRef]
40. Blalock, J.E. The syntax of immune-neuroendocrine communication. *Immunol. Today* **1994**, *15*, 504–511. [CrossRef]
41. Moreno-Ramos, O.A.; Lattig, M.C.; Barrios, A.F.G. Modeling of the hypothalamic-pituitary-adrenal axis-mediated interaction between the serotonin regulation pathway and the stress response using a Boolean Approximation: A novel study of depression. *Theor. Biol. Med. Model.* **2013**, *10*, 59. [CrossRef]
42. Kendall-Tackett, K.; Marshall, A.R.; Ness, K.E. Victimization, healthcare use, and health maintenance. *Fam. Viol. Sex. Assault Bull.* **2000**, *16*, 18–21.
43. Engel, G.L. The need for a new medical model: A challenge for biomedicine. *Science* **1977**, *196*, 129–136. [CrossRef]
44. Tricco, A.C.; Lillie, E.; Zarin, W.; O'Brien, K.K.; Colquhoun, H.; Levac, D.; Moher, D.; Peters, M.D.; Horsley, T.; Weeks, L. Prisma extension for Scoping Reviews (PRISMA-ScR): Checklist and Explanation. *Ann. Intern. Med.* **2018**, *169*, 467–473. [CrossRef] [PubMed]
45. Higgins, J.P.T.; Green, S. *Cochrane Handbook for Systematic Reviews of Interventions Version 5.1.0*; The Cochrane Collaboration: London, UK, 2011.

46. Horsley, S.; Dingwall, O.; Sampson, M. Checking reference lists to find additional studies for systematic reviews. *Cochrane Database Syst. Rev.* **2011**, *8*, MR000026. [CrossRef] [PubMed]
47. Beynon, R.; Leeflang, M.M.G.; McDonald, S.; Eisinga, A.; Mitchell, R.L.; Whiting, P.; Glanville, J.M. Search strategies to identify diagnostic accuracy studies in MEDLINE and EMBASE. *Cochrane Database Syst. Rev.* **2013**, *9*, MR000022. [CrossRef] [PubMed]
48. Moola, S.; Munn, Z.; Tufanaru, C.; Aromataris, E.; Sears, K.; Sfetc, R. Systematic reviews of etiology and risk. In *JBI Manual for Evidence Synthesis*; Aromataris., E., Munn, Z., Eds.; JBI: Adelaide, Australia, 2020. Available online: https://synthesismanual.jbi.global (accessed on 1 March 2023).
49. Parish, W.L.; Wang, T.; Laumann, E.O.; Pan, S.; Luo, Y. Intimate partner violence in China: National prevalence, risk factors and associated health problems. *Int. Fam. Plan Perspect.* **2004**, *30*, 174–181. [CrossRef] [PubMed]
50. Bonomi, A.E.; Anderson, M.L.; Rivara, F.P.; Thompson, R.S. Health outcomes in women with physical and sexual intimate partner violence exposure. *J. Womens Health* **2007**, *16*, 987–997. [CrossRef] [PubMed]
51. Hegarty, K.; Gunn, J.; Chondros, P.; Taft, A. Physical and social predictors of partner abuse in women attending general practice: A cross-sectional study. *Br. J. Gen. Pract.* **2008**, *58*, 484–487. [CrossRef]
52. Chartier, M.J.; Walker, J.R.; Naimark, B. Separate and cumulative effects of adverse childhood experiences in predicting adult health and health care utilization. *Child. Abuse Negl.* **2010**, *34*, 454–464. [CrossRef]
53. Vives-Cases, C.; Ruiz-Cantero, M.T.; Escriba-Aguir, V.; Miralles, J.J. The effect of intimate partner violence and other forms of violence against women on health. *J. Public Health* **2011**, *33*, 15–21. [CrossRef]
54. Williams, C.; Larsen, U.; McCloskey, L.A. The impact of childhood sexual abuse and intimate partner violence on sexually transmitted infections. *Violence Vict.* **2010**, *25*, 787–798. [CrossRef]
55. Eslick, G.D.; Koloski, N.A.; Talley, N.J. Sexual, physical, verbal/emotional abuse and unexplained chest pain. *Child. Abuse Negl.* **2011**, *35*, 601–605. [CrossRef]
56. Kelly, U.A.; Skelton, K.; Patel, M.; Bradley, B. More than military sexual trauma: Interpersonal violence, PTSD, and mental health in women veterans. *Res. Nurs. Health* **2011**, *34*, 457–467. [CrossRef] [PubMed]
57. Young, R.A.; Benold, T.; Whitham, J.; Burge, S. Factors influencing work interference in patients with chronic low back pain: A Residency Research Network of Texas (RRNet) study. *J. Am. Board. Fam. Med.* **2011**, *24*, 503–510. [CrossRef] [PubMed]
58. Gerber, M.R.; Fried, L.E.; Pineles, S.L.; Shipherd, J.C.; Bernstein, C.A. Posttraumatic stress disorder and intimate partner violence in a women's headache center. *Women Health* **2012**, *52*, 454–471. [CrossRef]
59. Saito, A.; Creedy, D.; Cooke, M.; Chaboyer, W. Effect of intimate partner violence on antenatal functional health status of childbearing women in Northeastern Thailand. *Health Care Women Int.* **2013**, *34*, 757–774. [CrossRef] [PubMed]
60. Sutherland, M.A.; Fantasia, H.D.; McClain, N. Abuse experiences, substance use, and reproductive health in women seeking care at an emergency department. *J. Emerg. Nurs.* **2013**, *39*, 326–333. [CrossRef]
61. Gelaye, B.; Do, N.; Avila, S.; Velez, J.C.; Zhong, Q.Y.; Sanchez, S.E.; Peterlin, B.L.; Williams, M.A. Childhood abuse, intimate partner violence and risk of migraine among pregnant women: An epidemiologic study. *Headache* **2016**, *56*, 976–986. [CrossRef]
62. Halpern, L.R.; Shealer, M.L.; Cho, R.; McMichael, E.B.; Rogers, J.; Ferguson-Young, D.; Mouton, C.P.; Tabatabai, M.; Southerland, P.G.; Gangula, P. Influence of intimate partner violence (IPV) exposure on cardiovascular and salivary biosensors: Is there a relationship? *J. Natl. Med. Assoc.* **2017**, *109*, 252–261. [CrossRef]
63. Lutgendorf, M.A.; Snipes, M.A.; O'Boyle, A.L. Prevalence and predictors of intimate partner violence in a military urogynecology clinic. *Mil. Med.* **2017**, *182*, e1634–e1638. [CrossRef]
64. England-Mason, G.; Casey, R.; Ferro, M.; MacMillan, H.L.; Tonmyr, L.; Gonzalez, A. Child maltreatment and adult multimorbidity: Results from the Canadian Community Health Survey. *Can. J. Public. Health* **2018**, *109*, 561–572. [CrossRef]
65. Grossi, P.K.; Bueno, C.H.; de Abreu Silva, M.A.; Pellizzer, E.P.; Grossi, M.L. Evaluation of sexual, physical, and emotional abuse in women diagnosed with temporomandibular disorders: A case-control study. *Int. J. Prosthodont.* **2018**, *31*, 543–551. [CrossRef]
66. Gucek, N.K.; Selic, P. Depression in intimate partner violence victims in Slovenia: A crippling pattern of factors identified in family practice attendees. *Int. J. Environ. Res. Public Health* **2018**, *15*, 210. [CrossRef] [PubMed]
67. Gunduz, N.; Erzican, E.; Polat, A. The relationship of intimate partner violence with psychiatric disorders and severity of pain among female patients with fibromyalgia. *Arch. Rheumatol.* **2019**, *34*, 245–252. [CrossRef] [PubMed]
68. Jovanovic, V.M.; Cankovic, S.; Milijasevic, D.; Ukropina, S.; Jovanovic, M.; Cankovic, D. Health consequences of domestic violence against women in Serbia. *Vojnosanit. Pregl.* **2020**, *77*, 14–21. [CrossRef]
69. Ali, T.S.; Sami, N.; Saeed, A.A.; Ali, P. Gynaecological morbidities among married women and husband's behaviour: Evidence from a community-based study. *Nurs. Open* **2021**, *8*, 553–561. [CrossRef] [PubMed]
70. Al Kendi, A.; Al Shidhani, N.; Al Kiyumi, M. Domestic violence among Omani women: Prevalence, risk factors and help-seeking behaviour. *East. Mediterr. Health J.* **2021**, *27*, 242–249. [CrossRef] [PubMed]
71. De Wet-Billings, N.; Godongwana, M. Exposure to intimate partner violence and hypertension outcomes among young women in South Africa. *Int. J. Hypertens.* **2021**, *2021*, 5519356. [CrossRef]
72. FitzPatrick, K.M.; Brown, S.; Hegarty, K.; Mensah, F.; Gartland, D. Physical and emotional intimate partner violence and women's health in the first year after childbirth: An Australian pregnancy cohort study. *J. Interpers. Violence* **2022**, *37*, NP2147–NP2176. [CrossRef]
73. Raphael, E.; Van Den Eeden, S.K.; Gibson, C.J.; Tonner, C.; Thom, D.H.; Subak, L.; Huang, A.J. Interpersonal violence and painful bladder symptoms in community-dwelling midlife to older women. *Am. J. Obstet. Gynecol.* **2022**, *226*, 230.e1–230.e10. [CrossRef]

74. Page, M.J.; McKenzie, J.E.; Bossuyt, P.M.; Boutron, I.; Hoffmann, T.C.; Mulrow, C.D.; Shamseer, L.; Tetzlaff, J.M.; Akl, E.A.; Brennan, S.E.; et al. The PRISMA 2020 statement: An updated guideline for reporting systematic reviews. *BMJ* **2021**, *372*, 71. [CrossRef]
75. Hassam, T.; Kelso, E.; Chowdary, P.; Yisma, E.; Mol, B.W.; Han, A. Sexual assault as a risk factor for gynaecological morbidity: An exploratory systematic review and meta-analysis. *Eur. J. Obstet. Gynecol. Reprod. Biol.* **2020**, *255*, 222–230. [CrossRef]
76. Matthews, K.A.; Woodall, K.L.; Allen, M.T. Cardiovascular reactivity to stress predicts future blood pressure status. *Hypertension* **1993**, *22*, 479–485. [CrossRef] [PubMed]
77. Turner, A.I.; Smyth, N.; Hall, S.J.; Torres, S.J.; Hussein, M.; Jayasinghe, S.U.; Ball, K.; Clow, A.J. Psychological stress reactivity and future health and disease outcomes: A systematic review of prospective evidence. *Psychoneuroendocrinology* **2020**, *114*, 104599. [CrossRef] [PubMed]
78. Lee, N.; Massetti, G.M.; Perry, E.W.; Self-Brown, S. Adverse childhood experiences and associated mental distress and suicide risk: Results from the Zambia violence against children survey. *J. Interpers. Violence* **2022**, *37*, NP21244–NP21265. [CrossRef]
79. Themelis, K.; Gillett, J.L.; Karadag, P.; Cheatle, M.D.; Giordano, N.A.; Balasubramanian, S.; Singh, S.P.; Tang, N.K. Mental defeat and suicidality in chronic pain: A prospective analysis. *J. Pain* **2023**, *in press*. [CrossRef] [PubMed]
80. Cherrier, C.; Courtois, R.; Rusch, E.; Potard, C. Self-esteem, social problem solving and intimate partner violence victimization in emerging adulthood. *Behav. Sci.* **2023**, *13*, 327. [CrossRef] [PubMed]
81. Bosch, J.; Weaver, T.L.; Arnold, L.D.; Clark, E.M. The impact of intimate partner violence on women's physical health: Findings from the Missouri Behavioral Risk Factor Surveillance System. *J. Interpers. Violence* **2017**, *32*, 3402–3419. [CrossRef] [PubMed]
82. Alhalal, E. Obesity in women who have experienced intimate partner violence. *J. Adv. Nurs.* **2018**, *74*, 2785–2797. [CrossRef]
83. Lopresti, A.L.; Drummond, P.D. Obesity and psychiatric disorders: Commonalities in dysregulated biological pathways and their implications for treatment. *Prog. Neuropsychopharmacol. Biol. Psychiatry* **2013**, *45*, 92–99. [CrossRef]
84. Wurtman, J.; Wurtman, R. The trajectory from mood to obesity. *Curr. Obes. Rep.* **2018**, *7*, 1–5. [CrossRef]
85. Okifuji, A.; Hare, B.D. The association between chronic pain and obesity. *J. Pain. Res.* **2015**, *8*, 399–408. [CrossRef]
86. Global Initiative for Asthma 2020. Available online: https://ginasthma.org/wp-content/uploads/2020/06/GINA-2020-report_20_06_04-1-wms.pdf (accessed on 5 April 2023).
87. Haczku, A.; Panettieri, R.A. Social stress and asthma: The role of corticosteroid insensitivity. *J. Allergy Clin. Inmmunol.* **2010**, *125*, 550–558. [CrossRef] [PubMed]
88. Subramanian, S.V.; Ackerson, L.K.; Subramanyam, M.A.; Wright, R.J. Domestic violence is associated with adult and childhood asthma prevalence in India. *Int. J. Epidemiol.* **2007**, *36*, 569–579. [CrossRef] [PubMed]
89. Rosenberg, S.L.; Miller, G.E.; Brehm, J.M.; Celedon, J.C. Stress and asthma: Novel insights on genetic, epigenetic, and immunologic mechanism. *J. Allergy Clin. Immunol.* **2014**, *134*, 1009–1015. [CrossRef] [PubMed]
90. Adler, E. *Erkrankungen durch Storfelder im Trigeminusbereich*; Fischer: Heidelberg, Germany, 1973.
91. Nakagawa, Y.; Yamada, S. Alterations in brain neural network and stress system in atopic dermatitis: Novel therapeutic interventions. *J. Pharmacol. Exp. Ther.* **2023**, *385*, 78–87. [CrossRef] [PubMed]
92. John, R.; Johnson, J.K.; Kukreja, S.; Found, M.; Lindow, S.W. Domestic violence: Prevalence and association with gynaecological symptoms. *BJOG* **2004**, *111*, 1128–1132. [CrossRef]
93. Letourneau, E.J.; Holmes, M.; Chasedunn-Roark, J. Gynaecologic health consequences to victims of interpersonal violence. *Womens Health Issues* **1999**, *9*, 115–120. [CrossRef]
94. Coker, A.L.; Smith, P.H.; Bethea, L.; King, M.R.; McKeown, R.E. Physical health consequences of physical and psychological intimate partner violence. *Arch. Fam. Med.* **2000**, *9*, 451–457. [CrossRef]
95. McCauley, J.; Kern, D.E.; Kolodner, K.; Dill, L.; Schroeder, A.F.; DeChant, H.K.; Ryden, J.; Bass, E.B.; Derogatis, L.R. The "battering syndrome": Prevalence and clinical characteristics of domestic violence in primary care internal medicine practices. *Ann. Intern. Med.* **1995**, *123*, 737–746. [CrossRef]

Disclaimer/Publisher's Note: The statements, opinions and data contained in all publications are solely those of the individual author(s) and contributor(s) and not of MDPI and/or the editor(s). MDPI and/or the editor(s) disclaim responsibility for any injury to people or property resulting from any ideas, methods, instructions or products referred to in the content.

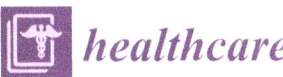

Article

Victimization and Perception of Abuse in Adolescent and Young Homosexual and Heterosexual Couples in Spain

Noelia Aguilera-Jiménez [1], Luis Rodríguez-Franco [2], Francisco Javier Rodríguez-Díaz [1], Jose Ramón Alameda-Bailén [3] and Susana G. Paíno-Quesada [3,*]

1. Department of Psychology, University of Oviedo, 33003 Oviedo, Spain; noelia.aguilera@dpee.uhu.es (N.A.-J.); gallego@uniovi.es (F.J.R.-D.)
2. Department of Personality, Assessment and Psychological Treatment, University of Seville, 41018 Seville, Spain; lurodri@us.es
3. Department of Clinical and Experimental Psychology, University of Huelva, 21071 Huelva, Spain; alameda@uhu.es
* Correspondence: sgpaino@uhu.es

Abstract: Currently, violence in adolescent and young couples has a significant social impact on young people's physical and psychological health. However, the study of violence in homosexual couples must also be addressed. This research analyzes the levels of violent victimization and the perception of abuse in both homosexual and heterosexual couples. Participants' ages ranged between 14 and 29 years ($M = 20.14$, $SD = 3.464$). We used The Dating Violence Questionnaire-Revised (CUIVNO-R), which was applied in two consecutive studies. The results indicate high levels of victimization, especially in the sample of homosexual participants. The scores generally show a low perception of couple violence but high victimization rates. The results of this study reveal the importance of the issue of violence in couples from minority groups and suggest that couple violence should not be understood as unidirectional, i.e., exclusively from men to women. These findings show the need for education in healthy relationships and consideration of different types of couples in these relationships.

Keywords: adolescent and young couple violence; homosexual couples; heterosexual couples; violent victimization; perception of abuse

1. Introduction

1.1. The Importance of the Study of Violence in Adolescent Couples and Young Homosexuals and Heterosexuals in the Spanish Context

In the Spanish context, the term to refer to intimate partner violence at the legislative level does not currently include violence between homosexual men or homosexual women or within the LGTBIQ+ collective. Therefore, official published data on these minority groups are scarce, and more so when it comes to adolescent couples and young homosexuals. Given the lack of data and the scarcity of findings related to the prevalence of violence in the latter group [1–3], our study analyzes this problem that affects adolescents' and young people's health and social and psychological well-being [4]. The main justification is that, so far, the investigations have adopted a heteronormative viewpoint [5]; that is, they have focused on heterosexual couples and, above all, on the one-directional violence of men towards women. However, it must be understood that violence can be present in any relationship; it can place anyone at risk and, just as in heterosexual couples, men and women with a homosexual orientation frequently suffer abusive behaviors of the same typologies: physical, psychological, and sexual abuse in the relationship [6–12].

Spain does not have official statistical data that specifically indicate the percentages of complaints from this community sample and, much less, from young couples. It must be added that it is especially complex for this group to request resources for help and guidance [3,13]. The lack of any description of how people manage these situations makes it impossible to develop effective and beneficial programs and resources for these minority groups [14], hence, the importance of this issue. Thus, it is necessary to know their characteristics to propose adapted responses based on better-adjusted violence-prevention guidance, the identification of the different ways of performing or suffering violence at these life stages, and—considering the current novelties—teaching relationships based on respect and attending to the well-being of the self and the other person.

1.2. Reference Terminologies for Intimate Partner Violence Research

It is essential to understand the terminology used in heterosexual and homosexual couple violence and in the LGTBIQ+ collective. On the one hand, we start with the term most frequently referenced: intimate partner violence (IPV), which, according to the World Health Organization [15] (p. 1), is understood as behavior within an intimate relationship that includes acts of physical aggression (slapping, hitting, or kicking), psychological abuse (intimidation, belittling, or continuous humiliation), forced sexual interactions, and controlling behaviors (isolation from family and friends, control of the partner's movements, and restriction of access to information or assistance). Another concept of interest is adolescent dating violence (DV), or Adolescent Dating Violence (ADV), or Teen Dating Violence (TDV). There are many definitions of these terms underlining the inclusion of intentional psychological, physical, and/or sexual abuse between people in a dating relationship [7]. DV has been studied for at least four decades [16]. In addition, the Centers for Disease Control and Prevention [17] adds that such abuse can be face-to-face or electronic, and Muñiz-Rivas et al. [18] indicate the importance of addressing online violence.

On the other hand, one of the terminologies to approach and better understand this neglected line of research regards violence performed in homosexual couples. In our context, the most consolidated term to refer to this is Intragender Violence (IV), which occurs in affective-sexual relationships between people of the same sex. It is the same as or similar to man-to-woman violence, with the intention of dominating and controlling the partner [19–21]. This stance generates discrepancy, as IV can refer to violence when one member of the couple is transgender, transsexual, intersexual, queer, or indeterminate, that is, couples within the LGTBIQ+ collective. In short, the term IV does not consider people or couples where one member belongs to the transsexual, transgender, or intersexual (TTI) collective and may be homosexual or heterosexual.

Understanding these terminologies requires identifying the differentiation offered in our legal context. Firstly, according to the Organic Law 1/2004 of December 28 on Comprehensive Protection Measures against Gender Violence [22], gender-based violence (or Intimate Partner Violence Against Women) is violence exercised only by the man to control or exercise power over the woman who is or has been a spouse or with whom he is or has been in a relationship with affective involvement, even without cohabitation. The exercise of power or the desire to control and dominate the other member of the affective relationship is shared in both GV (Gender-based Violence) and IV, but IV does not differentiate the sexes [19].

Finally, another confusing term is domestic violence (Law 27/2003, of July 31, regulating the order for the protection of victims of domestic violence) [23], which includes violence manifested in the family, previously or presently cohabitating, in which the victim can be either a man or a woman. However, although this excludes couples whose members are not spouses or cohabitants, it allows violence in homosexual couples to be legislated as domestic violence.

1.3. Contributions from the Literature on the Prevalence of Violence in Adolescent Couples and Young Homosexuals and Heterosexuals

Currently, IPV is a public health problem [8,9] affecting younger people in our society, as it begins at an early age [4,24]. Despite considering IV a global problem, this population has been neglected [25–27], highlighting the scarcity of published research, which is even more pronounced in our context.

The references on the prevalence of violence in homosexual couples reflect a high prevalence, with very significant percentages in the Spanish population [20,28]. This is also observed in the Latin American population, where both couple members are equally victims and perpetrators [29]. Other results are provided in the review by Edwards et al. [30], which indicated a higher prevalence among lesbian, gay, and bisexual people than among heterosexual people, consistent with other studies. Specifically, data on violence within homosexual couples show a prevalence range of 25.2–33.3% for men and 25–40.4% for women [31,32]. When specifying the typology, psychological violence reaches 63% for women and 60% for men [32]. Physical and sexual violence occurs among 44% of lesbians and 26% of gays [33]. Psychological victimization is the most frequent, followed by physical and sexual typologies [5,34]. In this regard, in Spain, Ortega [28], in his study on aggression in homosexual couples in a sample of young people aged 18 to 29, reports a prevalence of 13.09% for psychological violence, 4.57% for sexual violence, and 3.53% for physical violence, finding the highest rates of violent victimization in these minority groups for this age range.

Therefore, violence in this population seems to predispose it to a higher risk of mental health problems [25,35] and a higher probability of these individuals suffering violence in adulthood because they had suffered it in adolescence or youth [25,33]. There is also a lack of measures, evaluation instruments, and validations targeting these minorities, showing how urgent it is to create them [1].

1.4. Perception of Abuse in Adolescent Couples and Young Homosexuals and Heterosexuals

Finally, a little-studied but interesting phenomenon that has been neglected among these minorities is the perception of abuse by their partners, which has been studied in heterosexual couples [36–39]. This perception consists of a person's thoughts and cognitions when feeling abused by another person. In the Spanish population, many authors state that it is necessary to study not only the perception of being mistreated by one's partner but also the perception of stalking or the resulting feeling of fear, especially if the victim feels trapped in their relationship. This is closely connected to victimization through coercive behaviors or other more subtle forms of violence [37,38,40]. All this provides information about the characteristics of people who do not recognize or identify themselves as victims. Considering these dissonances, many researchers have highlighted the relevance of what is called "unperceived abuse-unperceived violence" or "technical abuse" [37–42]. It is interesting to note the results obtained by Gutiérrez Prieto et al. [43], who report that young people can recognize their partners' inappropriate actions, facilitating their perception of violent abuse regarding these behaviors.

Therefore, IPV should be addressed in a way that integrates all the different perspectives [44]. This would represent an advancement at the social, educational, and legal levels, considering the behaviors that, although just as illegal, are penalized differently. It is therefore essential to provide data that highlight this problem to adapt prevention and intervention projects for homosexual couples and the LGTBIQ+ collective.

We propose, as a general objective, to verify the levels of violent victimization and the perception of abuse in adolescent and young couples, both homosexual and heterosexual, to determine the scope of the problem in these minority groups (hereafter, we will use the terms heterosexual, homosexual, lesbian for couples of women, and gays for couples of men). The specific objectives are:

1. To analyze the prevalence of and differences in violent victimization according to sexual orientation (heterosexuals and homosexuals (gays and lesbians)) and sex.
2. To describe the perception of abuse (*feeling afraid or trapped in the relationship or feeling mistreated*) according to sexual orientation.

3. To verify the prevalence of victimization according to the existence of the perception of abuse based on sexual orientation and to observe a possible correspondence between victimization and levels of perception of abuse.

2. Method

2.1. Participants

The sample consists of 552 students of Compulsory Secondary Education, High school, Vocational training, and university from different provinces of Spain. Of them, 46% ($n = 254$) were female, and 54% ($n = 298$) were male, and their ages ranged between 14 and 29 years ($M = 20.14$, $SD = 3.464$). Of the participants, 156 (28.3%) reported having had a same-sex partner and 396 (71.7%) reported having had a partner of a different sex. Regarding those who reported having had same-sex partners, 48.7% ($n = 76$) were female, and 51.3% ($n = 80$) were male. Of the participants with different-sex partners, 44.9% ($n = 178$) were female, and 55.1% ($n = 218$) male. By level of education, 61.2% ($n = 338$) were pre-university students (Compulsory Secondary Education, High school, and Vocational training studies), and 38.6% ($n = 213$) were university students. Of the total sample, 90.2% responded *Yes* to the question "*Do you have a partner at this time?*" and 9.8% answered negatively. Finally, 21% were working. Concerning religion, 32.4% were not at all religious, 47.9% were moderately religious, and 24.8% were very religious.

Two groups were created for this research. On the one hand, we selected the cases where the participants indicated they had had or had a different-sex partner. This selection was exported to a different database, and two random samples of exact cases were extracted ($n = 198$). On the other hand, we selected the cases of participants who reported having had a same-sex partner ($n = 156$). Subsequently, the cases were entered into two different databases, resulting in the two studies analyzing 354 people (Study 1 and Study 2 (S1 and S2, respectively)).

2.2. Procedure

This research was carried out following the Declaration of Helsinki. As a large part of the sample was minors, compliance with the ethical criteria of working with minor participants was ensured. First, we arranged a meeting at the schools of Compulsory Secondary Education to explain the objectives of the research. After acceptance by the school directors, we collected the data. Data protection was guaranteed at all times. We provided all the groups with information about the usefulness and the purpose of the research to determine and describe the interpersonal dynamics within couple relationships. The groups were invited to participate voluntarily and received no compensation for their participation. Before completing the instruments, we obtained all the participants' informed consent and gave them the necessary instructions to complement the battery of instruments. This same procedure was carried out in the university centers.

This research used a non-probabilistic, intentional or judgment survey methodology because the sample was selected according to the requirements of the research goals.

2.3. Variables and Measurement Instruments

Sociodemographic characteristics. Sociodemographic information was collected about the participant and their partner: age, sex, level of education, income of the family nucleus, employment status, and religious beliefs.

Partner violence. We utilized the *Cuestionario de Violencia entre Novios, CUIVNO-R* [Dating Violence; Questionnaire] [2]. It comprises 20 items collecting information on victimization and perpetration of violence in young people's dating relationships. These items present behaviors or situations of abuse that can occur within the relationship, and their frequency is rated on a 5-point Likert scale ranging from 0 (*never*) to 4 (*almost always*). The CUIVNO-R offers 5 different forms of DV: *detachment, humiliation, coercion, physical violence, and sexual violence*. Detachment violence is evaluated, among others, via the following item: "your couple does not speak to you or leaves for several days, without any explanation, in order to show annoyance". Items regarding the other four DV forms include "violence through humiliation: your couple ridicules or insults you for the ideas you sustain"; "violence through coercion: your couple tests your love by setting up traps to see if you are cheating on your couple"; "sexual violence: you feel forced to comply certain sexual acts"; "physical violence: your couple has hit you". Internal consistency for the five scales ranges from 0.89 to 0.97 (Cronbach alpha), and for the total scale $\alpha = 0.98$. The internal consistency for the different scales of Study 1 ranged between 0.89 and 0.97 (Cronbach alpha) and for the total scale $\alpha = 0.98$. In Study 2, the indices of the different scales ranged from 0.90 to 0.98, and for the total scale $\alpha = 0.98$.

Perception of abuse. Following the requirements of the United Nations in 2015 [45] and because of the indications after the Istanbul Convention in 2011 [46], modifications were introduced in the Macro-Survey on Violence against Women (2015) [47], especially those related to the appropriateness of more accurately identifying forms of violence. Therefore, additional information was collected about whether the participant had experienced stalking (continuous or repeated harassment, following, spying) leading to fear of their partner. This indicator has been shown to be extremely effective in the latest official macro-survey carried out in Spain in 2019 on violence against women [40] and has been verified in previous empirical studies [42]. Through a second question, the participant was asked about their feeling of being trapped in the relationship to determine their subjective perception of the possibility of their being able to leave their affective relationship. Finally, we examined the perception or awareness of the situation of abuse. Specifically, there were 3 dichotomous questions with a *Yes* or *No* response: "*Do you feel or have you ever felt afraid of your partner?*", "*Do you feel or have you felt trapped in your relationship?*", and "*Have you felt mistreated in your relationship?*". The internal consistency for the total sample was $\alpha = 0.533$ (Study 1, $\alpha = 0.544$, and Study 2, $\alpha = 0.576$).

3. Statistical Analysis

The IBM SPSS statistical package, version 27, was used for data analysis. Descriptive statistics of the relevant variables of the study were conducted, assuming in all the analyses the criterion of "tolerance 0"; that is, violent behavior is considered to be present when any of the items that measure violent victimization is responded to with a value different from 0.

Prevalence of Violent Victimization in Adolescent Couples and Among Young Homosexuals and Heterosexuals. First, the typologies of violence according to the sexual orientation of each study group (heterosexual–homosexual) were analyzed. For this purpose, the level of victimization in the couple was calculated using the five subscales of CUIVNO-R (detachment, humiliation, coercion, and sexual and physical violence). Subsequently, we performed a Student's t contrast for independent samples and used the Bayes factor (BF) measures to determine the strength of the evidence of the differences. This same analysis was used considering the participants' sex and sexual orientation. We also analyzed the samples of participants who reported having had heterosexual partners and the couples of women (lesbians) and men (gays) who indicated having had homosexual partners. For this purpose, a repeated-measures analysis of variance (*ANOVA*) was carried out between the analyzed groups. Subsequently, the Bonferroni adjustment was calculated separately for the analysis of each group.

Perception of abuse in adolescent couples and among young homosexuals and heterosexuals. Secondly, we proceeded to describe the perception of abuse presented by the participants in the analyzed sample (feeling fear in the relationship, feeling trapped, or feeling mistreated). To this end, a descriptive frequency analysis was carried out to determine the percentage of participants who had answered any of the three questions affirmatively. Total scores and scores according to the sexual orientation of the sample were obtained. Subsequently, we calculated the difference in proportions for this analysis [48,49].

Violent Victimization and perception of abuse in adolescent couples and among young homosexuals and heterosexuals. We created two groups after the analyses to verify the correspondence between the victimization observed and the participants' perception of abuse. On the one hand, "Yes, Perception of Abuse" included the participants who had affirmatively answered any of the three questions on fear, entrapment, and abuse. The "No Perception of Abuse" comprised the participants who had answered all three questions negatively. In addition, the five factors of violence were transformed into dichotomous variables (0 = No Violence; 1 = Violence). Subsequently, "Total Violent Victimization" was obtained by adding the factors and transforming the variable to be dichotomous (0 = No Victimization; 1 = Victimization). After creating the groups, we determined the differences in their victimization rates of the five factors of violence of the CUIVNO-R and according to sexual orientation through chi-square (χ^2). Accordingly, we identified the people who presented indicators of violence that did not perceive them as such, as in other empirical studies [38,42,50].

4. Results

Below, the results of the two research studies are described and presented conjointly for more clarity. The sample of participants who indicated having had homosexual partners was used in the two studies.

Prevalence of violent victimization in adolescent couples and among young homosexuals and heterosexuals. In order to observe the prevalence of victimization and determine the differences in violent victimization (typologies of violence) between the two samples analyzed (according to sexual orientation), Student's t was performed to estimate the BF and calculate Cohen's effect size. The results (Table 1) indicate that homosexual couples obtained higher and statistically significant scores in both Studies 1 and 2. Physical violence (hitting, pushing, shaking, throwing objects, etc.) [S1: $t(346) = 38.35, p < 0.001, d = 2.88$; S2: $t(347) = 40.45, p < 0.001, d = 2.93$], detachment (disappearing, ceasing to talk to, and ignoring the partner's feelings) [S1: $t(347) = 29.06, p < 0.001, d = 2.61$; S2: $t(349) = 34.78, p < 0.001, d = 2.81$] and humiliation (insults and excessive criticism) [S1: $t(345) = 32.24, p < 0.001, d = 2.46$; S2: $t(346) = 32.81, p < 0.001, d = 2.45$] were the typologies with the greatest difference between the two samples, with effect sizes greater than 1, and the BF values reflect strong evidence of the obtained differences (BF = 0.000). To calculate the differences among heterosexual couples, gay couples, and lesbian couples, a one-factor ANOVA was performed. The corresponding repeated-measures ANOVA yielded significant group differences in the five types of violence identified in CUIVNO-R (Table 2). All typologies were significantly higher in the two groups of homosexual couples (gays and lesbians) than in the heterosexual group. However, when analyzing each group separately, the pairwise comparison with the Bonferroni adjustment showed significant differences between heterosexual couples and gay couples ($p = 0.000$) and between heterosexual couples and lesbian couples ($p = 0.000$) in both Study 1 and Study 2. On the other hand, we observed no significant differences between the groups of homosexual couples (gays and lesbians) except for sexual violence, which was significant in both studies [S1: $p = 0.003$; S2: $p = 0.002$].

Table 1. Violent Victimization in adolescent and young couples based on sexual orientation in Study 1 and Study 2.

Sexual Orientation/ Typologies of Violent Victimization		Heterosexuals		Homosexuals					
		n	$\bar{x}$	n	$\bar{x}$	BF	t	df	d
Detachment	S1	196	1.86	153	11.75	0.000	29.06 ***	347	2.61
	S2	198	1.12	153	11.75	0.000	34.78 ***	349	2.81
Humiliation	S1	197	0.70	150	11.29	0.000	32.24 ***	345	2.46
	S2	198	0.73	150	11.29	0.000	32.81 ***	346	2.45

Table 1. Cont.

Sexual Orientation/ Typologies of Violent Victimization		Heterosexuals		Homosexuals		BF	t	df	d
		n	x̄	n	x̄				
Coercion	S1	196	1.55	153	10.18	0.000	26.26 ***	347	2.23
	S2	198	0.85	153	10.18	0.000	31.38 ***	349	2.41
Sexual	S1	197	0.38	149	10.56	0.000	27.57 ***	344	2.04
	S2	196	0.24	149	10.56	0.000	28.60 ***	343	2.07
Physical	S1	197	0.36	151	12.85	0.000	38.35 ***	346	2.88
	S2	198	0.21	151	12.85	0.000	40.45 ***	347	2.93

Note. n: number of subjects; x̄: mean; BF: Bayes factor; t: Student's t; df: degrees of freedom; d: Cohen's d; S1: results Study 1; S2: results Study 2; *** $p < 0.001$.

Table 2. Repeated-measures analysis of variance of violent victimization of the groups in Study 1 and Study 2.

Sexual Orientation/ Typologies of Violent Victimization		Heterosexuals	Homosexuals		ANOVA
			Gay	Lesbians	
		x̄	x̄	x̄	F
Detachment	S1	1.86	11.57	11.93	421.89 ***
	S2	1.12	11.57	11.93	604.43 ***
Humiliation	S1	0.70	11.08	11.52	520.00 ***
	S2	0.73	11.08	11.52	538.33 ***
Coercion	S1	1.55	9.94	10.43	345.293 ***
	S2	0.85	9.94	10.43	493.20 ***
Sexual	S1	0.38	9.63	11.47	396.887 ***
	S2	0.24	9.64	11.47	427.33 ***
Physical	S1	0.36	12.55	13.14	737.357 ***
	S2	0.21	12.55	13.14	820.39 ***

Note. x̄: mean; ANOVA: repeated-measures ANOVA; F: F Test; S1: results Study 1; S2: results Study 2; *** $p < 0.001$.

Secondly, concerning the differences in violent victimization according to sex in both groups (homosexuals and heterosexuals), Table 3 shows statistically significant differences for all types of violence. Regarding the group of women, lesbians obtained the highest means, with the highest effect sizes in physical violence [S1: $t(163) = 24.95$, $p < 0.001$, $d = 2.87$; S2: $t(163) = 27.19$, $p < 0.001$, $d = 2.91$], violence due to detachment [S1: $t(162) = 19.58$, $p < 0.001$, $d = 2.58$; S2: $t(163) = 22.28$, $p < 0.001$, $d = 2.70$], and violence due to humiliation [S1: $t(159) = 21.36$, $p < 0.001$, $d = 2.37$; S2: $t(160) = 21.16$, $p < 0.001$, $d = 2.35$]. In men, the largest effect sizes were obtained for the typologies of physical violence [S1: $t(181) = 29.49$, $p < 0.001$, $d = 2.89$; S2: $t(182) = 29.94$, $p < 0.001$, $d = 2.92$] and detachment [S1: $t(183) = 21.42$, $p < 0.001$, $d = 2.65$; S2: $t(184) = 26.99$, $p < 0.001$, $d = 2.91$], followed by violence by humiliation [S1: $t(184) = 24.21$, $p < 0.001$, $d = 2.56$; S2: $t(184) = 25.39$, $p < 0.001$, $d = 2.57$] and coercion towards the partner [S1: $t(185) = 20.02$, $p < 0.001$, $d = 2.33$; S2: $t(185) = 23.30$, $p < 0.001$, $d = 2.52$], with gays again obtaining higher means. In addition, the Bayes factor ($BF = 0.000$) reflected strong evidence of the differences between homosexual and heterosexual women and men.

Table 3. Violent Victimization in adolescent and young couples based on sex and sexual orientation in Study 1 and Study 2.

Typologies of Violent Victimization/Sex/Sexual Orientation		n	$\bar{x}$ FHeterosexual	n	$\bar{x}$ FHomosexual	BF	t	df	d	n	$\bar{x}$ MHeterosexual	n	$\bar{x}$ MHomosexual	BF	t	df	d
Detachment	S1	88	1.74	76	11.93	0.000	19.58 ***	162	2.58	108	1.95	77	11.57	0.000	21.42 ***	183	2.65
	S2	89	1.24	76	11.93	0.000	22.28 ***	163	2.70	109	1.02	77	11.57	0.000	26.99 ***	184	2.91
Humiliation	S1	88	0.59	73	11.52	0.000	21.36 ***	159	2.37	109	0.79	77	11.08	0.000	24.21 ***	184	2.56
	S2	89	0.67	73	11.52	0.000	21.16 ***	160	2.35	109	0.78	77	11.08	0.000	25.39 ***	184	2.57
Coercion	S1	87	1.36	75	10.43	0.000	17.26 ***	160	2.16	109	1.70	78	9.93	0.000	20.02 ***	185	2.33
	S2	89	0.65	75	10.43	0.000	21.13 ***	162	2.33	109	1.02	78	9.94	0.000	23.30 ***	185	2.52
Sexual	S1	89	0.45	75	11.47	0.000	19.54 ***	162	2.16	108	0.32	74	9.63	0.000	19.77 ***	180	1.96
	S2	88	0.30	75	11.47	0.000	20.33 ***	161	2.19	108	0.20	74	9.64	0.000	20.44 ***	180	1.99
Physical	S1	89	0.36	76	13.14	0.000	24.95 ***	163	2.87	108	0.36	75	12.55	0.000	29.49 ***	181	2.89
	S2	89	0.17	76	13.14	0.000	27.19 ***	163	2.91	109	0.25	75	12.55	0.000	29.94 ***	182	2.92

Note. n: number of subjects; $\bar{x}$: mean; BF: Bayes factor; t: Student's t; df: degrees of freedom; d: Cohen's d; F: female; M: male; S1: results Study 1; S2: results Study 2; *** $p < 0.001$.

Perception of abuse in adolescent couples and among young homosexuals and heterosexuals. Figures 1 and 2 show that the feeling of being trapped in the relationship obtained the highest percentage for the total sample [S1: 25.40%; S2: 19.20%]. When analyzing the two groups, homosexual couples scored higher on all three questions in both studies. Moreover, significant scores were obtained when asking the participants about their feelings of entrapment in the relationship [S1: $p = 0.025$; S2: $p = 0.001$] and their fear of their partner [S2: $p = 0.001$] and feeling mistreated [S2: $p = 0.001$], although only in Study 2. Regarding the difference in proportions, the results indicated no significant differences between Study 1 and Study 2 in any of the responses concerning the perception of abuse (mistreatment, fear, and entrapment).

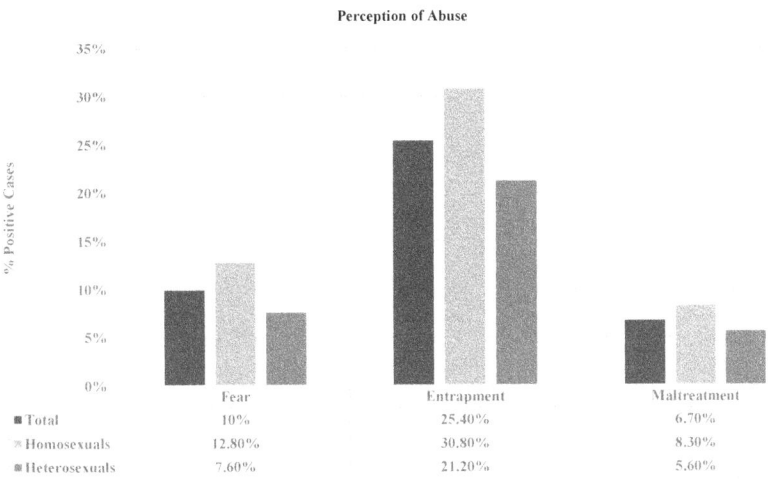

Figure 1. Percentages of positive cases of perception of abuse according to sexual orientation in the sample of Study 1.

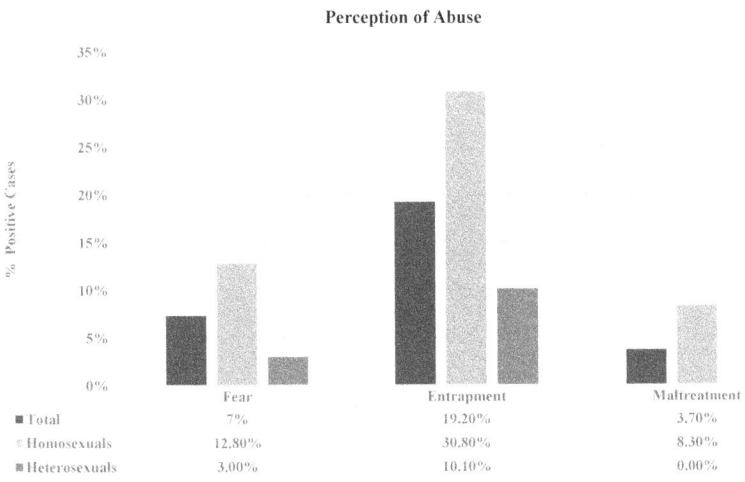

Figure 2. Percentages of positive cases of perception of abuse according to sexual orientation in the sample of Study 2.

Violent victimization and perception of abuse in adolescent couples and among young homosexuals and heterosexuals. Table 4 provides the percentages of perceived abuse ("Yes Perception of Abuse"/"No Perception of Abuse") in heterosexual and homosexual couples. Of the total sample, the percentage of participants who did not perceive abuse was higher in both studies [S1: n = 244 (68.90%); S2: n = 275 (77.70%)] than the percentage of those who perceived abuse [S1: n = 108 (30.50%); S2: n = 78 (22%)], with statistically significant differences [S1: χ^2 = 3.87, p = 0.032; S2: χ^2 = 31.61, p = 0.001]. We also observed higher violent victimization than non-victimization in the two studies. Specifically, we observed victimization scores ranging between 69.70% and 99.40% in contrast to non-victimization, which ranged between 0.60% and 30.30%. The presence of high levels of victimization and the high lack of perception of abuse are noteworthy. When inquiring about this, in both Studies 1 and 2, homosexual couples reached levels of victimization of 99.40%, whereas 63.50% of them perceived no abuse. Concerning the samples of heterosexual couples, in Study 1, 73.60% reported no perception of abuse, although 75.80% were victims of violence. In the case of Study 2, 88.90% did not perceive violence, although they presented victimization levels of 69.70%. Secondly, in the case of heterosexual couples, the chi-square revealed significant differences (in both studies) in all types of violence except for sexual and physical violence, which were nonsignificant in Study 2. The highest percentage of violence was observed in participants who had perceived abuse. However, this was not observed in the sample of homosexual couples, because only one case reported no victimization, whereas the remaining cases presented violent victimization with no differences among the typologies.

Finally, we examined the possible correspondence between the violent victimization observed in the two studies and the levels of perception of abuse. As seen in Figures 3 and 4, the high rates of violent victimization do not correspond to the perception of abuse indicated by the participants. Specifically, in homosexual couples (Studies 1 and 2), the percentage of victimization exceeded 90%, whereas the percentage of the perception of abuse did not exceed 31%. This mismatch also occurred among participants who reported having or having been heterosexual couples, although it was not as notable. In Study 1, violent victimization reached 59%, but the perception of violence only reached 21%. Consistent with the above, in Study 2, victimization also reached 44% compared to the 10% who had reported a perception of abuse. This highlights the invisibility of adolescents' and young people's suffering of violence.

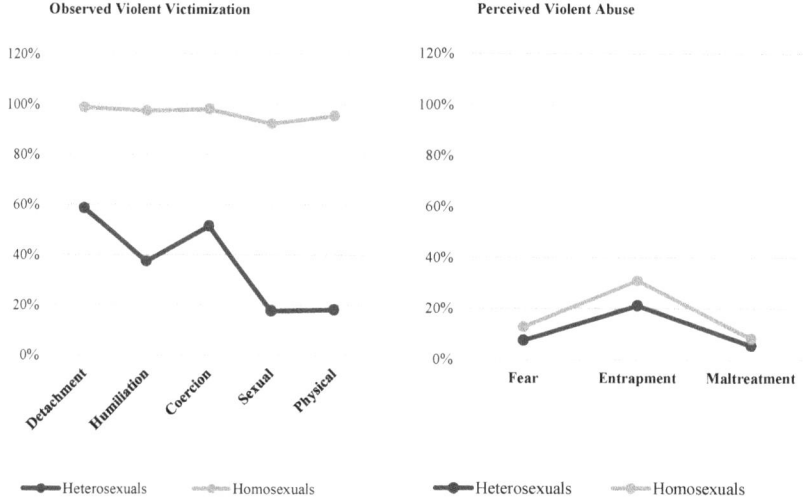

Figure 3. Visibility and invisibility of violent victimization and perception of abuse as a function of sexual orientation in Study 1.

Table 4. Levels of violent victimization and perception of abuse among homosexuals and heterosexuals in Study 1 and Study 2.

		Heterosexuals			Homosexuals		
		"Yes Perception of Abuse" n(%)	"No Perception of Abuse" n(%)	χ^2	"Yes Perception of Abuse" n(%)	"No Perception of Abuse" n(%)	χ^2
There is Victimization							
Detachment	S1	41(78.80%)	74(51.40%)	12.18 ***	59(100%)	97(98%)	1.15
	S2	16(72.70%)	71(40.30%)	8.33 **	59(100%)	97(98%)	1.15
Humiliation	S1	26(50%)	48(33.10%)	4.66 *	56(100%)	95(96%)	2.32
	S2	17(77.30%)	66(37.50%)	12.71 ***	56(100%)	95(96%)	2.32
Coercion	S1	41(78.80%)	60(41.40%)	21.50 ***	56(100%)	96(97%)	1.73
	S2	14(63.60%)	67(38.10%)	5.29 *	56(100%)	96(97%)	1.73
Sexual	S1	18(34.60%)	17(11.70%)	13.73 ***	54(96.4%)	89(89.90%)	2.13
	S2	7(31.80%)	28(15.90%)	3.40	54(96.4%)	89(89.90%)	2.13
Physical	S1	19(36.50%)	17(11.70%)	15.78 ***	55(98.2%)	93(93.90%)	1.52
	S2	5(22.70%)	18(10.20%)	2.98	55(98.2%)	93(93.90%)	1.52
Total Perception of Abuse	S1	52(26.30%)	145(73.20%)		56(35.9%)	99(63.50%)	
	S2	22(11.10%)	176(88.90%)		56(35.9%)	99(63.50%)	
		There is Victimization n(%)	No Victimization n(%)	χ^2	There is Victimization n(%)	No Victimization n(%)	
Total Violent Victimization	S1	150(75.80%)	48(24.20%)	16.14 ***	155(99.4%)	1(0.60%)	0.60
	S2	138(69.70%)	60(30.30%)	3.255	155(99.4%)	1(0.60%)	0.60

Note. N: number of subjects; %: percentage of subjects; χ^2: chi-square; S1: results Study 1; S2: results Study 2; F: female; M: male; * $p < 0.05$; ** $p < 0.01$; *** $p < 0.001$.

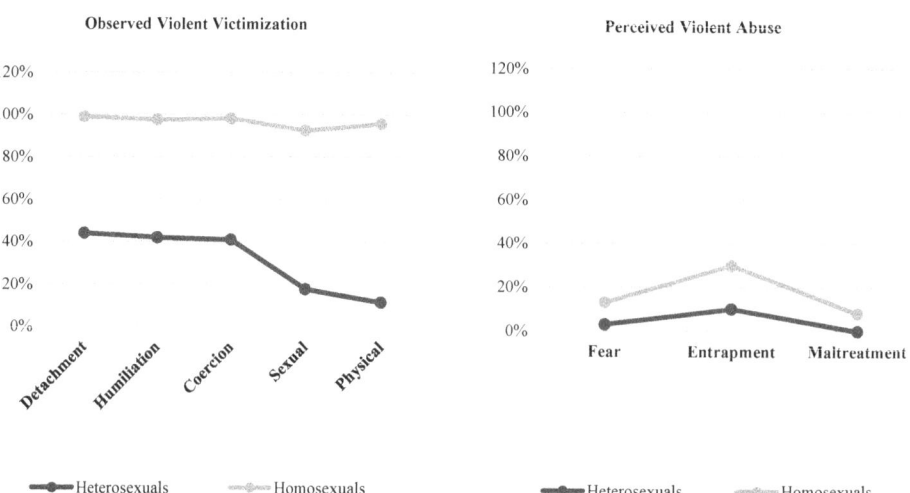

Figure 4. Visibility and invisibility of violent victimization and perception of abuse as a function of sexual orientation in Study 2.

5. Discussion

Violence is manifested in interpersonal relationships; specifically, this study shows that violence in homosexual couples is a problem of the same dimension as violence in heterosexual couples. Therefore, it is essential to ensure its adequate legal treatment considering all existing dimensions, like IPV. According to the approach and the findings, this study provides novel information on the extent of the problem of IPV in vulnerable groups. In light of our results, we underline the high frequency of IPV among both heterosexuals and homosexuals, showing the need to be aware that violence can appear in any interpersonal relationship. Consequently, we must educate youth in having care and respect for the other person and provide sexual education and sufficient information so that young people can identify the indicators of violence, which can affect their physical, mental, and social health.

First, based on the principle of "zero tolerance", our results are consistent with other studies carried out in Spain and Latin America finding comparable rates of victimization among both homosexuals and heterosexuals—although higher among the former [20,28,29]—as well as with the data published in other countries, such as that of Edwards et al. [30]. Among homosexuals, physical victimization stands out, followed by other types of violence, such as psychological or unperceived violence; that is, detachment (disappearing or not talking or ignoring the partner's feelings) and humiliation (insults or criticism of the partner). When comparing our findings on homosexual couples with other investigations, there are some discrepancies; in particular, a discrepancy is observed in the order in which the typologies of violence are presented. That is, physical violence, detachment, and humiliation of the partner are more frequent in our results than sexual violence and coercion, which are also present but with lower rates. In contrast, other studies, such as that of Ortega [28], report that in samples of adolescents and young people (from 14 to 29 years old), psychological violence obtains the highest percentage, followed by sexual and physical violence. The same is true of the results of Walters et al. [32], where psychological violence was more frequent than physical violence, or the results obtained by Martín-Storey [33], where physical and sexual violence predominated among these minorities. This is not observed in heterosexuals, whose members are mostly victims of violence due to detachment, coercion, and humiliation, in coherence with the findings of other studies where psychological violence prevails [10,37–39,42].

Despite this controversy, the analyses show the different types of violent victimization within couple relationships, highlighting the results among homosexuals [5,31,32,34]. In young heterosexual relationships, we confirm the high prevalence of psychological violence performed and suffered both by males and females, with detachment, coercion, and humiliation being common [10,38].

Another relevant finding of this study is the differences in all the typologies of violence (both in heterosexual and homosexual couples) as a function of the participants' sex. Females suffer more physical victimization, detachment, and humiliation, mostly in homosexual couples. On the other hand, males repeat the typologies of physical violence, detachment, and humiliation, also adding coercion. Therefore, this shows that victimization can affect anyone. Hence, limiting the roles of female victims and male aggressors implies ignoring the existing reality because victimization affects a large part of the population [51]. Thus, the predominance of humiliating one's partner, especially in homosexual couples, reveals what the LGTBIQ+ collective refers to when they talk about the threat of "coming out of the closet" or "outness". This threat is aimed at controlling or retaining the other member of the relationship by threatening them with society's ridicule and contempt. This phenomenon suffered by these minorities promotes tension and stress in the relationship dynamic, turning it negative [52]. The findings of violence exercised through coercion, which is more predominant in males, are consistent with the meta-analysis of Spencer et al. [53], which reports that this typology of violence is a risk factor among young men. On the other hand, according to the data on physical violence, victimization in homosexual relationships, regardless of sex, is striking, following research indicating that males are perpetrators of physical violence and females of mild physical violence [38,54].

Summing up, we can state that our adolescent and young populations are immersed in violent relationships, with a tendency to perpetuate and normalize the dynamics of conflictive relationships [55], and two issues are essential: (1) violence at this stage can become violence in adulthood [24,25,33]; and (2) violence puts the physical and mental health of our younger population at risk [4,8,9].

Thirdly, with the aim of complying with the recommendations of the European Council [46] and the Macro-Survey on Violence against Women of 2015 and 2019 [40,47], we investigated the different ways of experiencing violence. We found percentages ranging from 3.70% to 25.40%, with homosexual couples reporting feeling these indicators to a greater extent. In particular, we emphasize that the feeling of being trapped in a relationship is the most frequent in the adolescent and young populations. This information is relevant for the study and future prevention as it can indicate emotional dependence on one's partner, which correlates with negative coping in conflictive situations [41]. On the other hand, we found that fear of one's partner presents percentages around 7–10%, indicating the possible existence of concealed cases of partner violence. These data are similar to those published by the 2019 Macro-Survey [40], suggesting that 13.90% of females aged 16 and older feared their partners. The perception of abuse in the relationship is shown to have the lowest prevalence. This is probably due to the difficulty of recognizing oneself as someone who is in an abusive or violent situation [39]. Similarly, this may also be due to the reductionist interpretation of psychological violence or unperceived violence, which poses a clear risk because it is considered a predictor of the partner's physical violence [38–42,56].

On the other hand, regarding the third objective, we verified an evident lack of perception of abuse and high levels of victimization. These data generate alarm and should be addressed in prevention programs, and we highlight that of the total sample of homosexual couples, only one person was not victimized. Finally, from a global point of view, the couples in this research had difficulty in perceiving abuse because the percentage of "Perception of Abuse" was small (S1: 30.5%; S2: 22%) in contrast to the high levels of victimization observed. The non-perception of violence in heterosexual couples has already been detected in different studies [38–43]. A higher percentage of homosexual couples than heterosexual couples fails to recognize suffering violence as such; like other research, the data indicate a limited level of awareness of homosexual violence [36].

All the above leads us to consider that anyone can suffer violence within a couple relationship [6]. Although there are indeed differences between homosexual and heterosexual couples, this only indicates that victimization also exists within these couples, and there may even be a lack of perception of abusive acts. Thus, violence is present in our affective relationships and continues to be a worldwide problem affecting the public health of our adolescents and young people globally [8,9,11,12]. These results serve to propose changing the unique view that risk is only present in heterosexual couples because there is risk among men and women who have same-sex partners and in relationships where one member is transsexual, intersexual, queer, or indeterminate; in short, this risk exists for people who have interpersonal relationships with other people.

6. Limitations

Regarding the main limitations of this research, we point out the sample size. It would be interesting to increase it to generalize the results of violent victimization for our context. Samples of people with different sexual orientations or gender identities should be obtained to determine the differences due to maturational development according to age. The second limitation refers to the absence of data on the perpetration of violence. Integrating this variable would enable us to know if the victim is also an aggressor; that is, we could analyze the bi-directionality of violence, mainly in homosexual couples.

7. Conclusions

In conclusion, there is a need for changes in public and social policies so that the victims of violence have social resources. Regardless of whether they are heterosexual or of the LGTBIQ+ collective, this issue is still a social emergency. Neither the LGTBIQ+ nor the heterosexual populations seek IPV-related support services. In the former case, this is because of the barriers to receiving care [57], and, in the latter case, because of the difficulty of perceiving their relationship as abusive and, therefore, themselves as victims [38].

From this point of view, violence in homosexual couples must be considered a problem with the same dimensions as violence in heterosexual couples, and, therefore, resources must be adapted to the needs of this minority group [26]. In other words, it is necessary to apply social and egalitarian measures, educational measures that promote respect, and legal measures in which the system endorses and performs comprehensive evaluations where both members of the couple (victims and aggressors) are assessed without establishing differences. In short, defending the existence of other types of violence does not imply making gender differences invisible but rather avoids limiting violence exclusively to gender differences [44].

Finally, regarding future lines of research, we confirm the importance of addressing this area of prevention, given the results of different investigations on unperceived violence and high levels of violent victimization, with the justification of violence as a risk factor for victimization [58]. In this way, we can identify the indicators present in conflictive situations where inadequate coping strategies are implemented, generating abusive behaviors that are fully normalized. Therefore, we should continue to perform informative prevention, talk to young people, and conceptualize all the possible present and future situations they may encounter so that they can respond adequately for their well-being and that of others. Another critical point recommended by the United Nations [45] is the need to ask women if they have ever felt afraid of their current partner or their ex-partners. Our contributions indicate that not only should one ask women about fear, but exploring the feeling of entrapment and mistreatment in anyone within an interpersonal relationship is also relevant. Secondly, psychological proposals should be offered to create judicial measures of violence in homosexual couples to increase their sense of security and society's protection towards these minority groups. Thirdly, there is a need for a working approach comparable to that used with heterosexual couples that analyzes not only the level of victimization but also the level of perpetration of violence, that is, that addresses bi-directional violence in same-sex couples, as noted above in the limitations. Finally, we should not ignore the need to develop specific and effective action plans because bi-directional violence may be a common pattern in relationships [38].

Author Contributions: Conceptualization, N.A.-J., L.R.-F., F.J.R.-D., J.R.A.-B. and S.G.P.-Q.; data curation, N.A.-J., L.R.-F., F.J.R.-D., J.R.A.-B. and S.G.P.-Q.; formal analysis, N.A.-J., L.R.-F., F.J.R.-D., J.R.A.-B. and S.G.P.-Q.; investigation, N.A.-J., L.R.-F., F.J.R.-D., J.R.A.-B. and S.G.P.-Q.; methodology, N.A.-J., L.R.-F., F.J.R.-D., J.R.A.-B. and S.G.P.-Q.; project administration, N.A.-J., L.R.-F., F.J.R.-D., J.R.A.-B. and S.G.P.-Q.; resources, N.A.-J., L.R.-F., F.J.R.-D., J.R.A.-B. and S.G.P.-Q.; software, N.A.-J., L.R.-F., F.J.R.-D., J.R.A.-B. and S.G.P.-Q.; supervision, N.A.-J., L.R.-F., F.J.R.-D., J.R.A.-B. and S.G.P.-Q.; validation, N.A.-J., L.R.-F., F.J.R.-D., J.R.A.-B. and S.G.P.-Q.; visualization, N.A.-J., L.R.-F., F.J.R.-D., J.R.A.-B. and S.G.P.-Q.; writing—original draft, N.A.-J., L.R.-F., F.J.R.-D., J.R.A.-B. and S.G.P.-Q.; writing—review and editing, N.A.-J., L.R.-F., F.J.R.-D., J.R.A.-B. and S.G.P.-Q. All authors have read and agreed to the published version of the manuscript.

Funding: This work was supported by the European Regional Development Funds (European Union and Principality of Asturias) through the Science, Technology and Innovation Plan (AYUD/2021/51411) and the State Research Agency of the Ministry of Economic Affairs and Digital Transformation (MCI-21-PID2020-114736GB-100).

Institutional Review Board Statement: The protocol of the study was not evaluated by the Ethics Committee of our university because it did not include invasive procedures; it did not include collection, use, or storage of biological samples from subjects; nor did it include collection, use, or storage of genetic information from participants. The study was carried out in Spain. Following the current Spanish legislation, approval from the Ethics Committee is mandatory only when a study protocol includes any of these procedures.

Informed Consent Statement: Informed consent was obtained from all the participants involved in the study.

Data Availability Statement: The data reported here are available at request by scientific community members.

Acknowledgments: The authors wish to thank all the participants for their collaboration in completing this research.

Conflicts of Interest: The authors of this article declare that they have no conflict of interest.

References

1. Barrientos, J.; Rodríguez-Carballeira, A.; Escatín, J.; Longares, L. Violencia en parejas del mismo sexo: Revisión y perspectivas actuals [Violence in same-sex couples: Review and current perspectives]. *Rev. Argent. Clín. Psicol.* **2016**, *XXV*, 289–298. Available online: https://www.redalyc.org/pdf/2819/281948416008.pdf (accessed on 15 February 2023).
2. Rodríguez-Díaz, F.J.; Herrero, J.; Rodríguez-Franco, L.; Bringas-Molleda, C.; Paíno-Quesada, S.G.; Pérez, B. Validation of Dating Violence Questionnaire-R (DVQ-R). *Int. J. Clin. Health Psychol.* **2017**, *17*, 77–84. [CrossRef] [PubMed]
3. Rojas-Solís, J.L.; Rojas, I.; Meza, R.N.; Villalobos, A. Violencia de parejas gays y en hombres que tienen sexo con hombres: Una revisión sistemática exploratoria [Violence by gay partners and men who have sex with men: An exploratory systematic review]. *Rev. Crim.* **2021**, *63*, 173–186. Available online: http://www.scielo.org.co/pdf/crim/v63n1/1794-3108-crim-63-01-173.pdf (accessed on 8 April 2023).
4. Barroso-Corroto, E.; Cobo-Cuenca, A.I.; Laredo-Aguilera, J.A.; Santacruz-Salas, E.; Pozuelo-Carrascosa, D.P.; Rodríguez-Cañamero, S.; Martín-Espinos, N.M.; Carmona-Torres, J. Dating violence, violence in social networks, anxiety and depression in nursing degree students: A cross-sectional study. *J. Adv. Nurs.* **2022**, *79*, 1451–1463. [CrossRef]
5. Gómez, F.; Barrientos, J.; Guzmán, M.; Cárdenas, M.; Bahamondes, J. Violencia de pareja en hombres gay y mujeres lesbianas chilenas: Un estudio exploratorio [Intimate partner violence in Chilean gay men and lesbian women: An exploratory study]. *Interdisciplinaria* **2017**, *34*, 57–72. Available online: https://www.redalyc.org/pdf/180/18052925004.pdf (accessed on 25 January 2023).
6. Loinaz, I.; Ortiz-Tallo, M.; Sánchez, L.M.; Ferragut, M. Clasificación multiaxial de agresores de pareja en centros penitenciarios [Multiaxial classification of partner aggressors in prisons]. *Int. J. Clin. Health Psychol.* **2011**, *11*, 249–268. Available online: http://www.aepc.es/ijchp/articulos_pdf/ijchp-379.pdf (accessed on 5 December 2022).
7. Taquette, S.R.; Monteiro, D.L.M. Causes and consequences of adolescent dating violence: A systematic review. *J. Inj. Violence Res.* **2019**, *11*, 137–147. [CrossRef]
8. García-Díaz, V.; Lana-Pérez, A.; Fernández-Feito, A.; Bringas-Molleda, C.; Rodríguez-Franco, L.; Rodríguez-Díaz, F.J. Actitudes sexistas y reconocimiento del maltrato en parejas jóvenes [Sexist attitudes and recognition of abuse in young couples]. *Aten. Prim.* **2018**, *50*, 398–405. [CrossRef]

9. Heyman, R.E.; Kogan, C.S.; Foran, H.M.; Burns, S.C.; Slep, A.M.S.; Wojda, A.K.; Keeley, J.W.; Rebello, T.J.; Reed, G.M. A case-controlled field study evaluating ICD-11 proposals for relational problems and intimate partner violence. *Int. J. Clin. Health Psychol.* **2018**, *18*, 113–123. [CrossRef]
10. Aguilera-Jiménez, N.; Rodríguez-Franco, L.; Rohlfs Domínguez, P.; Alameda Bailén, J.R.; Paíno-Quesada, S.G. Relationships of adolescent and young couples with violent behaviors: Conflict resolution strategies. *Int. J. Environ. Res. Public Health* **2021**, *18*, 3201. [CrossRef]
11. Ferrer-Pérez, V.A.; Bosch-Fiol, E. El Género en el Análisis de la Violencia Contra las Mujeres en la Pareja: De la "Ceguera" de Género a la Investigación Específica del Mismo [Gender in the Analysis of Intimate Partner Violence against Women: From Gender "Blindness" to Gender-Specific Research]. *Anuario de Psicología Jurídica* **2019**, *29*, 69–76. [CrossRef]
12. Rubio-Garay, F.; López-González, M.A.; Carrasco, M.A.; Amor, P.J. Prevalencia de la violencia en el noviazgo: Una revisión sistemática [Prevalence of dating violence: A systematic review]. *Pap. Psicol.* **2017**, *38*, 135–147. [CrossRef]
13. Rojas-Solís, J.L.; Guzmán-Pimentel, M.; Jiménez-Castro, P.; Martínez-Ruiz, L.; Flores-Hernández, B.G. La violencia hacia los hombres en la pareja heterosexual: Una revisión de revisions [Violence against men in heterosexual couples: A review of reviews]. *CyS* **2019**, *44*, 57–70. [CrossRef]
14. Kubicek, K.; McNeeley, M.; Collins, S. "Same-sex relationship in a straight world": Individual and societal influences on power and control in young men's relationships. *J. Interpers. Violence* **2015**, *30*, 83–109. [CrossRef] [PubMed]
15. World Health Organization. *Comprender y Abordar la Violencia Contra las Mujeres. Violencia Infligida por la Pareja 2013 [Understanding and Addressing Violence against Women. Intimate Partner Violence 2013]*; Washington, DC, USA, 2013; Available online: https://apps.who.int/iris/bitstream/handle/10665/98816/WHO_RHR_12.36_spa.pdf?sequence=1 (accessed on 17 September 2022).
16. Exner-Cortnes, D. Chapter13-Measuring adolescent dating violence. In *Adolescent Dating Violence: Theory, Research, and Prevention*; Wolfe, D.A., Temple, J.R., Eds.; Academic Press: Cambridge, MA, USA, 2018; pp. 315–340. [CrossRef]
17. Centers for Disease Control and Prevention. Preventing Teen Dating Volence. What Is Teen Dating Violence? 2021. Available online: https://www.cdc.gov/violenceprevention/intimatepartnerviolence/teendatingviolence/fastfact.html (accessed on 9 December 2022).
18. Muñiz-Rivas, M.; Suárez-Relinque, C.; Estévez, E.; Povedano-Díaz, A. Víctimas de violencia de pareja en la adolescencia: El papel del uso problemático de las redes sociales virtuales, la soledad y el clima familia [Victims of intimate partner violence in adolescence: The role of problematic use of virtual social networks, loneliness and family climate]. *Anu. Psicol.* **2023**, *39*, 127–136. [CrossRef]
19. Aldarte; Centro de Atención a Gays, Lesbianas y Transexuales. Por los Buenos Tratos en las Relaciones Lésbicas y Homosexuales. Informe para la Inclusión de la Perspectiva LGTB en los Planteamientos Sobre Violencia de Género: Propuestas para el Debate ["For Good Treatment in Lesbian and Homosexual Relationships". Report for the Inclusion of the LGBT Perspective in Approaches to Gender Violence: Proposals for Discussion]. 2012. Available online: https://www.aldarte.org/comun/imagenes/documentos/BUENOSTRATOS.pdf (accessed on 13 October 2022).
20. Aldarte; Centro de Atención a Gays, Lesbianas y Transexuales. Estudio Sobre Violencia Intragénero. Informe Encuesta Violencia intragénero ["Study on Intragender Violence. Intragender Violence Survey Report"]. 2010. Available online: http://www.aldarte.org/comun/imagenes/documentos/informeencuestaviolenciaintragenero.pdf (accessed on 5 February 2023).
21. Rodríguez Otero, L.M.; Lameiras, M.; Carrera, M.V. Violencia en parejas gays, lesbianas y bisexuales: Una revisión sistemática 2002–2012 [Violence in gay, lesbian and bisexual couples: A systematic review]. *Comunitaria* **2017**, *13*, 49–71. [CrossRef]
22. Ley Orgánica 1/2004, de 28 de diciembre, de Medidas de Protección Integral contra la Violencia de Género. BOE de 29 de Diciembre de 2004 [Measures of Integral Protection against Gender-Based Violence. BOE of 29 December 2004]. Available online: https://www.boe.es/eli/es/lo/2004/12/28/1/con (accessed on 19 November 2022).
23. Ley 27/2003, of July 31, Reguladora de la Orden de Protección de las Víctimas de la Violencia Doméstica. BOE, número 183, de 1 de agosto de 2003 [Regulator of the Order of Protection of Domestic Violence Victims. BOE, Number 183, of 1 August 2003]. Available online: https://www.boe.es/eli/es/l/2003/07/31/27 (accessed on 19 November 2022).
24. Carrascosa, L.; Cava, M.J.; Buelga, S. Perfil psicosocial de adolescentes españoles agresores y víctimas de violencia de pareja [Psychosocial profile of Spanish adolescent aggressors and victims of intimate partner violence]. *Univ. Psychol.* **2018**, *17*, 1–10. [CrossRef]
25. Gillum, T.L. Adolescent dating violence experiences among sexual minority youth and implications for subsequent relationship quality. *Child. Adolesc. Soc. Work. J.* **2017**, *34*, 137–145. [CrossRef]
26. Laskey, P.; Bates, E.A.; Taylor, J.C. A systematic literature review of intimate partner violence victimization: An inclusive review across gender and sexuality. *Aggress. Violent. Behav.* **2019**, *47*, 1–11. [CrossRef]
27. Trombetta, T.; Rollè, L. Intimate partner violence perpetration among sexual minority people and associated factors: A systematic review of quantitative studies. *Sex. Res. Social. Policy* 2022, published online. [CrossRef]
28. Ortega, A. Agresión en parejas homosexuales en España y Argentina: Prevalencias y heterosexismo [Aggression in homosexual couples in Spain and Argentina: Prevalences and heterosexism]. Ph.D. Thesis, Universidad Complutense de Madrid, Madrid, Spain, 2014. Available online: https://eprints.ucm.es/id/eprint/28389/1/T35737.pdf (accessed on 13 March 2022).
29. Romero-Méndez, C.A.; Gómez, M.J.; Romo-Tobón, R.J.; Rojas-Solís, J.C. Violencia en la pareja en jóvenes mexicanos del mismo sexo: Un estudio exploratorio [Intimate partner violence in Mexican same-sex youth: An exploratory study]. *ACADEMO* **2020**, *7*, 136–147. [CrossRef]

30. Edwards, K.M.; Sylaska, K.M.; Neal, A.M. Intimate partner violence among sexual minority population: A critical review of the literature agenda for future research. *Psychol. Violence* **2015**, *5*, 112–121. [CrossRef]
31. Taylor, N.T.B.; Herman, J.L. Intimate Partner Violence and Sexual Abuse among LGBT People: A Review of Existing Research. The Williams Institute. 2015. Available online: https://williamsinstitute.law.ucla.edu/wp-content/uploads/IPV-Sexual-Abuse-Among-LGBT-Nov-2015.pdf (accessed on 12 June 2022).
32. Walters, M.L.; Chen, J.; Breiding, M.J. *The National Intimate Partner and Sexual Violence Survey (NISVS): 2010 Findings on Victimization by Sexual Orientation*; National Center for Injury Prevention and Control, Centers for Disease Control and Prevention: Atlant, GA, USA, 2013. Available online: https://www.cdc.gov/violenceprevention/pdf/nisvs_sofindings.pdf (accessed on 16 March 2022).
33. Martin-Storey, A. Prevalence of dating violence among sexual minority youth: Variation across gender, sexual minority identity and gender of sexual partners. *J. Youth Adolesc.* **2015**, *44*, 211–224. [CrossRef] [PubMed]
34. Barrientos, J.; Escartín, J.; Longares, L.; Rodríguez-Caballeira, A. Sociodemographic characteristics of gay and lesbian victims of intimate partner psychological abuse in Spain and Latin America. *Int. J. Soc. Psychol.* **2018**, *33*, 240–274. [CrossRef]
35. Rodríguez, J.G.; Momeñe, J.; Olave, L.; Estévez, A.; Iruarrizaga, I. La Dependencia Emocional y la Resolución de Conflictos en Heterosexuales, Homosexuales y Bisexuals [Emotional Dependence and Conflict Resolution in Heterosexuals, Homosexuals, and Bisexuals]. *RED* **2019**, *44*, 59–79. Available online: https://www.aesed.com/upload/files/v44n1_art3.pdf (accessed on 11 April 2022).
36. Bornstein, D.R.; Fawcett, J.; Sullivan, M.; Senturia, K.D.; Shiu-Thornton, S. Understanding the experiences of lesbian, bisexual and trans survivors of domestic violence: A qualitative study. *J. Homosex.* **2006**, *51*, 159–181. [CrossRef]
37. López-Cepero, J.; Lana, A.; Rodríguez-Franco, L.; Paíno, S.G.; Rodríguez-Díaz, F.J. Percepción y etiquetado de la experiencia violenta en las relaciones de noviazgo juvenil [Perception and labeling of violent experience in youth dating relationships]. *Gac. Sanit.* **2015**, *29*, 21–26. [CrossRef]
38. Paíno-Quesada, S.G.; Aguilera-Jiménez, N.; Rodríguez-Franco, L.; Rodríguez-Díaz, F.J.; Alameda-Bailén, J.R. Adolescent conflict and young adult couple relationships: Directionality of violence. *Int. J. Psychol. Res.* **2020**, *13*, 36–48. [CrossRef]
39. López-Cepero, J.; Rodríguez-Franco, L.; Rodríguez-Díaz, F.J.; Bringas-Molleda, C.; Paíno, S.G. Percepción de la victimización en el noviazgo de adolescentes y jóvenes españoles [Perception of victimization in the dating relationships of Spanish adolescents and young people]. *Rev. Iberoam. Psicol. Salud.* **2015**, *6*, 64–71. [CrossRef]
40. Delegación del Gobierno para la Violencia de Género. Subdirección General de Sensibilización, Prevención y Estudios de la Violencia de Género. Macroencuesta de Violencia contra la Mujer 2019 [Macro-Survey of Violence against Women 2019]. Ministerio de Igualdad; 2020. Available online: https://violenciagenero.igualdad.gob.es/violenciaEnCifras/macroencuesta2015/pdf/Macroencuesta_2019_estudio_investigacion.pdf (accessed on 20 May 2022).
41. Martín, B.; Moral, M.V. Relación entre dependencia emocional y maltrato psicológico en forma de victimización y agresión en jóvenes [Relationship between emotional dependence and psychological abuse in the form of victimization and aggression in young people]. *Rev. Iberoam. Psicol. Salud.* **2019**, *10*, 75–89. [CrossRef]
42. Rodríguez-Franco, L.; López-Cepero, L.; Rodríguez-Díaz, F.J.; Bringas Molleda, C.; Estrada Pineda, C.; Antuña Bellerín, M.A.; Quevedo-Blasco, R. Labeling dating abuse. Undetected abuse among Spanish adolescents and young adults. *Int. J. Clin. Health Psychol* **2012**, *12*, 55–67. Available online: https://www.redalyc.org/pdf/337/33723707004.pdf (accessed on 26 April 2022).
43. Gutiérrez Prieto, B.; Bringas-Molleda, C.; Tornavacas Amado, R. Autopercepción de maltrato y actitudes ante la victimización en las relaciones interpersonales de pareja [Self-perception of abuse and attitudes towards victimization in interpersonal relationships]. *Anu. Psicol.* **2022**, *52*, 220–227.
44. Echeburúa, E. Sobre el papel del género en la violencia de pareja contra la mujer. Comentario a Ferrer-Pérez y Bosch-Fiol, 2019 [On the role of gender in intimate partner violence against women. Comment to Ferrer-Pérez y Bosch-Fiol, 2019]. *Anu. Psicol. Jurídica* **2019**, *29*, 77–79. [CrossRef]
45. United Nations. Directrices para la producción de estadísticas sobre la violencia contra la mujer: Encuesta estadística. [Guidelines for the Production of Statistics on Violence against Women. Statistical Surveys]. 2015. Available online: https://oig.cepal.org/sites/default/files/directrices_estadisticas_violencia_contra_la_mujer.pdf (accessed on 1 June 2022).
46. Comisión Europea. Convenio del Consejo de Europa sobre Prevención y Lucha contra la Violencia contra las Mujeres y la Violencia Doméstica. Estambul, Turquía [Council of Europe Convention on the Prevention and Fight against Violence against Women and Domestic Violence]. Istanbul, Turkey, 2011; 11v. Available online: https://rm.coe.int/1680462543 (accessed on 10 September 2022).
47. Delegación Gobierno para la Violencia de Género. Macroencuesta de Violencia contra la Mujer 2015 [Macro-Survey of Violence against Women 2015]. Ministerio de Sanidad, Servicios Sociales e Igualdad. Centro de Publicaciones; 2015. Available online: https://violenciagenero.igualdad.gob.es/violenciaEnCifras/estudios/colecciones/pdf/Libro_22_Macroencuesta2015.pdf (accessed on 23 March 2023).
48. Moore, D.S.; McCabe, G.P. *Introduction to the Practice of Statistics*, 4th ed.; Freeman, W.H., Ed.; EEUU: New York, NY, USA, 2003.
49. Pryce, G. *Inference and Statistics in SPSS: A Course for Business and Social Science*; GeeBeeJey: Glasgow, UK, 2005.
50. Rodríguez-Franco, L.; Gracia, C.; Juarros-Baterretxea, J.; Fernández-Suárez, A.; Rodríguez-Díaz, F.J. Agresores generalistas y especialistas en violencia de parejas jóvenes y adolescentes: Implicaciones en la implementación de los programas de prevención [Generalist and specialist batterers in teen and young dating violence: Implications for the development of prevention programs]. *Acción Psicol.* **2017**, *14*, 1–16. [CrossRef]

51. Rojas-Solís, J.L.; Romero-Méndez, C.A. Violencia en el noviazgo: Análisis sobre su direccionalidad, percepción, aceptación, consideración de gravedad y búsqueda de apoyo [Dating violence: Analysis of its directionality, perception, acceptance, consideration of severity and search for support]. *Health Addict.* **2022**, *22*, 132–151. [CrossRef]
52. Feinstein, B.A.; McConnell, E.; Dyar, C.; Mustanski, B.; Newcomb, M.E. Minority stress and relationship functioning among young male same-sex couples: An examination of actor-partner interdependence models. *J. Consult. Clin. Psychol.* **2019**, *86*, 416–420. [CrossRef]
53. Spencer, C.; Toews, M.; Anders, K.; Emanuels, S. Risck Markers for physical teen dating violence perpetration: A meta-analysis. *Trauma Violence Abuse* **2019**, *22*, 619–631. [CrossRef]
54. Gracia-Leiva, M.; Puente-Martínez, A.; Ubillos-Landa, S.; Páez-Rovira, D. La violencia en el noviazgo (VN): Una revisión de meta-análisis [Dating violence (DV): A meta-analysis review]. *An. Psicol.* **2019**, *35*, 300–313. [CrossRef]
55. Bonache, H.; Ramírez-Santana, G.; González-Méndez, R. Conflict resolution styles and teen dating violence. *Int. J. Clin. Health Psychol.* **2016**, *16*, 276–286. [CrossRef]
56. Juarros-Baterretxea, J.; Overall, N.; Herrero, J.; Rodríguez-Díaz, F.J. Considering the effect of sexism on psychological intimate partner violence: A study with imprisoned men. *Eur. J. Psych. Appl. Legal Context.* **2019**, *11*, 61–69. [CrossRef]
57. Scheer, J.R.; Martín-Storey, A.; Baams, L. Help-seeking barriers among sexual and gender minority individuals who experience intimate partner violence victimization. In *Intimate Partner Violence and the LGBT+ Community*; Russell, B., Ed.; Springer Nature: Cham, Switzerland, 2020; pp. 139–158. [CrossRef]
58. Galdo-Castiñeiras, J.A.; Hernández-Morante, J.J.; Morales-Moreno, I.; Echevarría-Pérez, P. Educational intervention to decrease justification of adolescent dating violence: A comparative quasi-experimental study. *Healthcare* **2023**, *11*, 1156. [CrossRef] [PubMed]

Disclaimer/Publisher's Note: The statements, opinions and data contained in all publications are solely those of the individual author(s) and contributor(s) and not of MDPI and/or the editor(s). MDPI and/or the editor(s) disclaim responsibility for any injury to people or property resulting from any ideas, methods, instructions or products referred to in the content.

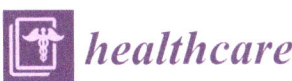

Review

Barriers Faced by Australian and New Zealand Women When Sharing Experiences of Family Violence with Primary Healthcare Providers: A Scoping Review

Jayamini Chathurika Rathnayake, Nadirah Mat Pozian, Julie-Anne Carroll * and Julie King

School of Public Health and Social Work, Faculty of Health, Queensland University of Technology, Kelvin Grove Campus, Victoria Park Road, Kelvin Grove, QLD 5069, Australia; sra.rathnayake@connect.qut.edu.au (J.C.R.); nadirah.matpozian@hdr.qut.edu.au (N.M.P.); j.macknight-king@qut.edu.au (J.K.)
* Correspondence: jm.carroll@qut.edu.au

Abstract: Despite the Australian Government's attempts to reduce domestic violence (DV) incidences, impediments within the social and health systems and current interventions designed to identify DV victims may be contributing to female victims' reluctance to disclose DV experiences to their primary healthcare providers. This scoping review aimed to provide the state of evidence regarding reluctance to disclose DV incidents, symptoms and comorbidities that patients present to healthcare providers, current detection systems and interventions in clinical settings, and recommendations to generate more effective responses to DV. Findings revealed that female victims are reluctant to disclose DV because they do not trust or believe that general practitioners can help them to solve their issues, and they do not acknowledge that they are in an abusive relationship, and are unaware that they are in one, or have been victims of DV. The most common symptoms and comorbidities victims present with are sleep difficulties, substance use and anxiety. Not all GPs are equipped with knowledge about comorbidities signalling cases of DV. These DV screening programs are the most prominent intervention types within Australian primary health services and are currently not sufficiently nuanced nor sensitive to screen with accuracy. Finally, this scoping review provides formative evidence that in order for more accurate and reliable data regarding disclosure in healthcare settings to be collected, gender power imbalances in the health workforce should be redressed, and advocacy of gender equality and the change of social structures in both Australia and New Zealand remain the focus for reducing DV in these countries.

Keywords: domestic violence; primary healthcare; general practitioners; female victims; nurses; midwives

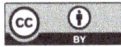

1. Introduction

Domestic violence (DV) is characterised as a series of behaviours used by a perpetrator to obtain or maintain power and authority over an intimate partner in any relationship, as well as over children and/or siblings with whom they share a similar household or a domestic relationship [1,2]. The most prominent forms of gender-based violence are intimate partner violence, rape, sexual assault and stalking [3,4]. DV is regarded as a violation of women's rights and has emerged as a major and urgent public health issue [5–8]. Eradicating violence against women was included in the United Nations' Millennium Development Goals (in 2000) as well as in the Sustainable Development Goal 5 (Gender Equality) (in 2015) [6,9].

Extant findings demonstrate that DV adversely affects women's health, overall functioning and well-being—in the short and/or the long term (e.g., quality of life) [5–12]. According to the US Department of Health and Human Services (USDHHS) [13], short-term impacts of DV include injuries, bleeding, miscarriages, unplanned pregnancies, sexually transmitted infections and insomnia. The USDHHS [13] further states that the long-term effects of DV include arthritis, asthma, sleeping problems, migraines, headaches, stress, depression and chronic pain. Furthermore, the immediate and ongoing impacts of DV on women's health have been identified in a variety of areas, including mental health issues and physical damage, such as bruises, cuts, teeth and gum damage, skin lesions, stillbirths and head injuries. Studies reveal the signs of DV perpetration include harmful behaviours against children and pets, as well as the use of unsafe driving to instil fear and coercion [4,14,15].

Among these complications, the most concerns expressed by Australian women were mental well-being issues [3,11]. DV is significantly associated with mental health disorders) and is a leading cause of death, disability or illness [3,16]. Additionally, DV impacts individuals' financial status and contributes to poverty, especially homelessness. According to Dillon et al. [17], there is an increasing correlation between DV and homelessness, particularly among women and children. This evidence corroborates with Mission Australia [18], which stated that in 2018 and 2019, 80,000 women sought professional homelessness support services.

Prevalence of DV in Australia

Although DV is regarded as a critical national health and welfare issue [19] and the most unspeakable crime in Australia [7], there has been an unprecedented rise in violence and harassment against women over the last three decades [3,20]. According to the Australian Bureau of Statistics Personal Safety Survey 2016, an estimated one in six women (over the age of 15) experienced sexual or physical violence from a current or former cohabiting partner, with women being were more likely to encounter violence from a known individual and in their home [20,21]. Nevertheless, the magnitude of DV incidence remains unknown [22].

Between 2014 and 2015, a woman was killed every nine days by her intimate partner in Australia [19]. In 2017, more than 11,000 women between the age of 15 and 34 experienced DV or sexual harassment [19]. Women are more likely to become victims during their reproductive years [23–25]. According to Gartland et al. [24], 20–30% of women suffered physical or mental abuse 1–4 years postpartum. A meta-synthesis study reveals that women aged 45 and above are also at risk of family violence, which may lead to the risk of homelessness in old age [7,26]. There is also a higher risk of family and DV during major crises, such as epidemics and natural disasters [27,28]. Moreover, increases in the number of DV incidents and the frequency of victims visiting primary healthcare services intensify the burden on medical practitioners and frontline healthcare providers [29].

The Australian Government and healthcare sector, both at federal and state levels, are striving to take immediate and decisive action on behalf of victims [30–32]. As a widespread service provider, the healthcare sector can provide high-quality healthcare and ensure supportive environments are in place both to enable victims to disclose DV lived experiences and to help victims and survivors overcome their issues [9,33]. Despite these efforts, numerous impediments remain within the current settings (both health and social systems) and interventions [10,34]. These impediments may lead female victims to be reluctant in disclosing their lived experiences of DV to primary healthcare workers or general practitioners (GPs) [10].

While the devastating impact of DV on women and those that they care for is well documented, and the extent of the problem across both Australia and New Zealand carefully tracked, the phenomenon cannot be either accurately measured nor treated if women remain reluctant to disclose the problem to frontline healthcare providers. Further, while community workers in the DV space tend to be the 'safe spaces' female DV sufferers go to for assistance, there is a call for greater trust building amongst these same women and GPs in particular. Further, there is an established need for clinicians to be better trained at detecting reluctance to share DV experiences with them in private appointments. This scoping review aimed to collate the relevant literature in a bid to generate a cohesive, evidence-based narrative around barriers for reporting DV within clinical settings in a bid to provide this information to those who need it most.

We aimed to provide an updated and focused review of the barriers female victims face in revealing DV experiences to primary healthcare professionals in the clinical setting and private appointments with GPs. This review generated a summary of (i) the reasons why DV victims do not disclose to GPs and primary healthcare professionals, (ii) symptoms and comorbidities that patients present to healthcare providers, (iii) current detection approaches and quality of interventions in the clinical setting, and (iv) finally provides recommendations to generate more effective responses to DV to clinicians specifically.

2. Materials and Methods

2.1. Scoping Review Research Questions and Objectives

This study aims to answer the following research questions: (i) What are the reasons DV victims do not disclose to GPs and primary healthcare professionals? (ii) What are the comorbidities and symptoms that DV patients present with? and (iii) what are the current methods of detection and interventions in clinical settings. The objective was to combine the findings to provide recommendations to both researchers and clinicians regarding more effective responses to DV.

2.2. Data Sources and Search Strategy

A scoping methodology was used to conduct the review and identify the results. Several search strategies were developed during the process to identify the relevant studies. Four primary databases were used, including CINHAL (nursing and allied health database), PsycINFO, Embase and PubMed. The term 'domestic violence' was mainly used to identify articles using the synonyms of 'family violence', 'intimate partner violence', 'battered women' and 'domestic violence victims'. The phrase 'domestic violence' and its synonyms (with a truncation mark) were used along with phrases such as 'barriers to express', 'barriers to reveal', 'enablers to reveal' and 'motivations to reveal' to identify the relevant articles. Boolean operators were used to expand the results.

2.3. Eligibility Criteria

This scoping review included all study designs, including qualitative, quantitative and mixed-method studies. It focused on Australian and New Zealand studies, given that New Zealand has a similar public health service to Australia. Only full-text articles in English were considered and included in the review.

2.4. Exclusion Criteria

All editorials, letters to the editor, newspaper articles, thesis reviews, dissertations and articles from low- and middle-income countries were excluded from the scoping review. Additionally, studies that discussed substance use and DV and postpartum depression and DV were not considered. Figure 1 displays the process used, including the inclusion and exclusion criteria.

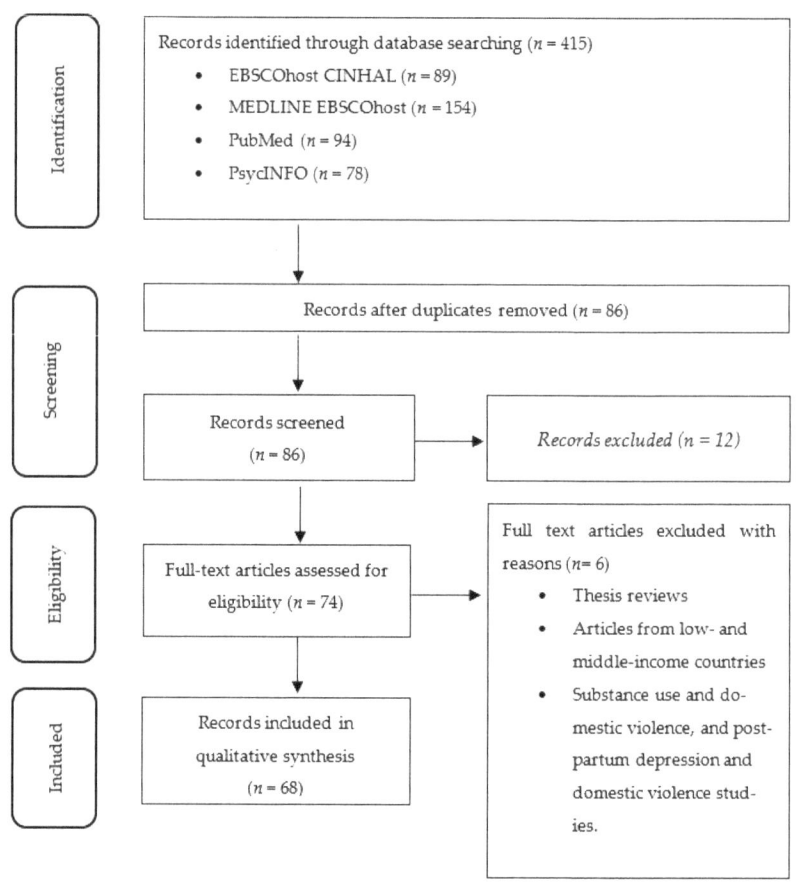

Figure 1. The flow diagram for the selection process and reasons for exclusion of studies.

3. Results

3.1. Why DV Victims Do Not Disclose to GPs and Other Primary Health Professionals

GPs are the primary healthcare workers who identify DV most frequently during private appointments through assessments and diagnostic processes [35]. There is still much debate and discussion about who discloses (both voluntarily and unwillingly) DV experiences to GPs and reports DV side effects (e.g., addictions, insomnia and wounds in various stages of health) but not the abuse itself [35–37]. Studies by O' Doherty et al. [34], Meuleners et al. [22] and Hegarty et al. [10] report that most DV victims do not trust their GPs as a professional to whom they can disclose their DV experiences and related illnesses and injuries. Further, victims do not accept their GPs as a solution to solve DV-related issues [22,34,38]. Generally, DV victims have reported that they view GPs solely as clinical health practitioners, rather than as counsellors or professional supporters to whom they would reveal such violence [34]. Hence, most victims seek GPs only to treat their injury, wounds or physical harm; they do not want to obtain psychological or social support [22].

Victims also do not disclose these injuries as DV cases or as part of the abuse to their GPs. DV victims are more likely to disclose injuries or physical harm as accidents or falls rather than abuse [39]. The critical case is that abused women do not like to acknowledge that they are in an abusive relationship and are or had been victims of DV [34,39,40]. Some women were unaware that they had become a victim of a perpetrator or that the violence was part of the DV phenomenon [10,39]. Consequently, despite being able to recognise DV symptoms, it is a complex and difficult task for primary healthcare providers to provide support to victims who do not recognise and acknowledge that they are in unhealthy relationships and are at risk of ongoing and worsening abuse [39]. Overall, there is a significantly low rate of DV disclosure to GPs during clinical appointments; even when DV is identified, it remains challenging to discuss with the victims and even more difficult to intervene with sustained success [20,36–38,40].

3.2. What Symptoms and Comorbidities Do Patients Present to Healthcare Providers?

Evidence shows the prevalence of DV is common among women who visit GPs [36,37,40,41]. However, women tend not to present their DV experiences or symptoms as symptoms of abuse, whether directly or overtly. Instead, the DV experiences are made visible through many other indirect ways. The most common visible ways of DV and family violence symptoms being reported to GPs include minor injuries at different stages of healing, sleep issues, low self-esteem and other mental health problems [5,10,42].

Sleep difficulty is one of the most common problems among women who experience acts of violence [42–44]. However, this symptom is often associated with other women's health issues, thus making it difficult to ascertain whether or not women are experiencing violence, assault or abuse. Many women who suffer from DV request prescriptions for sleep medication with synchronous symptoms of depression, anxiety and a desire or compulsion to self-harm [42]. It is challenging for GPs to initiate conversations about violence that women may face from their partner [42].

Mental health issues or psychological factors are key symptoms raised during GP visits by women who experience DV [34,42,45]. Most DV victims, whether they identify as such or not, attend their general practice regularly with comorbidities of mental and physical health issues [5,10,46]. Included studies reveal that female DV victims experience numerous mental health problems [3,23,34,45,47]. Generally, DV victims have very poor mental health and struggle to cope or function in everyday life [3,5,10]. Victims' poor emotional well-being has a significant impact on their decision-making processes. For example, women visit GPs in a state of panic or anxiety, often having trouble communicating clearly at these times [34,45]. Women frequently want to seek professional support, yet they attempt to avoid doing so by convincing themselves that other people would perceive them as bad wives or partners [23,34]. Some women tend to think that they can manage DV situations by themselves; others think that the situations are temporary and will eventually resolve themselves, or that their abuser was going through a 'bad phase' or having a bad day [23,34]. Some victims "Dr shop" to avoid disclosing the real cause of their injuries and illnesses by seeing multiple GPs for a particular incident [22]. These mental factors often compound within the victims, thus preventing them from revealing their DV experiences.

Fear is a highly common characteristics among patients who visit GPs and other health services as the result of DV [5,10,47]. It has long been established that fear is a key barrier for women communicating abuse to primary healthcare providers [39]. Many women are unwilling to disclose what has happened, and most victims attempt to minimise the harmful incident [39]. Fears identified include fear of consequences from their partner, fear of more violence, fear of losing their partner and fear that they will not be believed [10,47].

Fear is a common psychological factor that patients experiencing DV exhibit, and while some of the causes of fear have been noted, an additional fear pertains to financial dependency [10]. According to the literature, victims' financial situation is a crucial deciding factor in their willingness or confidence to disclose abuse [23,39,45]. Women who are financially dependent on their partners are afraid that they will be unable to survive without a source of income. Many abusers will work to ensure financial dependency as part of their abuse, coercion and control strategies. The abusers may do this directly by not allowing their partner to work, damaging their chances of working or forbidding contraception so that unplanned pregnancies make continued employment difficult [48–50]. Women's income and motherhood status are also factors that prevented them from reporting the abuse to GPs or even leaving their partners [39,45].

3.3. Detection and Intervention in the Clinical Setting

The majority of female psychiatrists revealed that dealing with DV was not their responsibility or obligation [47]. DV is an issue that community health workers should handle rather than primary healthcare professionals or psychiatrists [47]. Male psychiatrists indicated that psychiatrists did not assist in identifying DV victims, but the appointment of a specific staff member would [47]. In addition, male psychiatrists reported that listening to and treating and dealing with female DV victims was a difficult and uncomfortable job because they felt guilty about the situations of their female patients [7,47].

GP centres, in theory, are intended to provide a safe and confidential way to disclose violence and abuse incidents [51]. These settings have unique characteristics for early abuse identification and are equipped in many ways to prevent DV through effective interventions and referral mechanisms [40]. Patient awareness of their GP's availability, their trust in the healthcare practitioners and the potential feelings of comfortableness are the advantages of these settings as areas with great potential for effective DV intervention [40,51]. Evidence shows that a patient's trust in GPs and GP centres is higher than in other types of primary health service providers. Patients also intended to use GP services more regularly than other types of health and social services, making them potent contact points for initiating DV conversations, such as what DV is and how to get help to escape abuse [10]. For these reasons, these clinical settings have been recognised as potentially efficacious settings for DV screening and identifying interventions [34] Many health professionals and health organisations recommend screening programs as an early-stage intervention method for readdressing and stopping DV and family violence [5,10].

The WEAVE randomised control trial (RCT) was one of the first studies to evaluate a DV screening-related program among women, with implications and suggested potential improvements for GP-based interventions [10,34,38]. The study helped to identify several ways of screening implementation and aiding effective intervention [34,38]. In addition, the MOVE study was the first RCT to determine the effectiveness of identifying intimate partner violence in a community-based nursing setting [32,52]. The MOVE was an intervention with a resource guide about intimate partner violence [32]. This study can be considered an effective step because it provided health practitioners in the clinical setting with relevant resources. According to the final MOVE intervention, the final results had no impact on regular reporting of DV cases or screening in referrals [32]. On the one hand, findings showed the same participants were involved in the intervention as a negative impact and noted a significant increase only in safety planning as a positive impact [32]. However, the study shed new light on self-completion checklists, which were effective in the clinical setting and contributed to a slight difference in establishing pathways to discuss DV experiences [32]. Overall, nursing-based models have proven to be effective in primary healthcare settings. However, the interventions or screening programs are required to be consistent with a victim's safety planning, rather than simply asking direct questions to detect DV or family violence [32]. Safety of the victims who disclose abuse remains paramount during any screening or intervention activity, regardless of its point of administration or delivery [32].

Primary health professionals utilise numerous screening tools. The most popular screening tools are Hurt, Insult, Threaten and Scream [53]. Generally, this involves the screener asking the primary health service user questions during a screening process [34,54,55]. The screener has the opportunity to identify DV victims if they reveal their real condition, but most of the time, the victims do not do so [54,56]. In addition to the basic screening tools, brief health screening items, written or electronic identification methods, and in-person meetings have been reviewed and recognised as effective tools for reaching out to DV victims [36,52]. Risk assessment is another way of identifying family violence. It is mandatory in most primary health settings to implement a screening process before conducting a risk assessment [55]. During the risk assessment process, practitioners have the opportunity to ask more detailed questions [10]. Routine screening is another common strategy used in the primary healthcare setting [32,36]. Routine screening includes regular physical examination check-ups for skin conditions, sexually transmitted diseases and the eyes, as well as blood pressure levels [57]. Another approach that has shown some success in assisting women suffering from abuse is the 'case finding' or inquiry approach [32]. The case-finding approach can be applied in any DV situation, but healthcare workers should have relevant training to handle cases [32]. Social work professionals are more likely to use the case-finding approach, and in this scenario, public health professionals must work together with them. This method can map out victims' personal experience in analysing DV situations [58–60].

Unfortunately, the reality at the pragmatic level differs from the theory [54,56,61]. Various complications have been found in screening programs, though screening is considered as a recognised way of identifying and preventing individuals from becoming victims or perpetrators. Moreover, screening for complex social phenomena in GP centres demonstrates a very low or limited data yield overall [32,36,52].

The screening process has several issues that needed to be rectified by the responsible authorities. Common claims include not interviewing in a private setting or space, having too many staff members involved in the screening process, the screener not being the same gender or race as the victims, the presence of the victim's partner and age gaps between the victim and screener [54,56,61]. However, there is currently insufficient data or evidence to draw decisive conclusions about the effectiveness and potential for screening DV within GP practices and clinics [54,56,61]. The quality and outcome of DV screening programs and intervention processes depend on the timing and nature of the delivery of the questions by the healthcare provider to the patient [52].

Research has highlighted the complications and barriers to successful DV intervention and screening by GPs [5,34,36]. Firstly, the research acknowledges how profound the breakthrough can be for the patients and women who were disclosing their experiences for the first time. Due to the various reasons and fears that prevent women from revealing their living conditions, a GP's chances of detection remain low overall. Establishing the necessary trust to reveal such experiences was profound and difficult for any health service provider to achieve [34,36]. Secondly, to be effective and safe, GP-based interventions in primary care settings should consider the different types and severity of abuse faced by women [10]. A common or universal general intervention is not feasible for the whole target population who have experienced DV. Nuanced responses and referrals are required to make discerning insights about the specific type of treatment and support the best matches for the experiences of each unique woman. Thirdly, there are still concerns that GP-based screenings and individual case data collection efforts do not always provide a complete and accurate account of the specific characteristics of the type and severity of harm [10]. One of the most frequently used data collection methods, self-reporting, has been discovered to have an inherent bias [5,10]. Response bias is a general complication within this type of data collection method [5,62]. Addressing all the characteristics of this highly diverse and vulnerable target population through a GP centre or individual clinic visits alone is a daunting and complex goal to achieve [34]. More research is needed on screening tools and strategies for the timing and nature of their delivery and administration if GPs are to achieve greater success in their efforts to assist victims and survivors to escape and fully recover from DV [38].

Finally, screening as an intervention tool for identifying DV remains questionable. It has several biases when used in the primary healthcare setting. It is therefore worthwhile to consider what is needed to generate more effective responses to DV in the primary healthcare setting.

3.4. Recommendations for More Effective Responses to DV in Primary Healthcare Settings

The literature widely acknowledges that improvements in the primary healthcare setting are much needed if they are to be better and more trusted places for victims of DV and other domestic abuse to seek assistance [37,40]. Beyond the internal reviews, evaluations of the screening tools and an increased capacity for GPs to be able to respond to patients suffering from DV are needed. DV experts and other community health service providers have weighed in to provide insights into how primary healthcare providers can better respond to this highly sensitive, diverse and complex social phenomenon.

When considering the macro level of the healthcare setting, one meaningful suggestion is that feminist-driven approaches need to be implemented in a primary healthcare setting to tackle gender imbalances in the clinical health context [63]. Literature suggests DV is a highly cultural and gendered issue that can be seen in many social structures [64]. This significant debate concerning power imbalances also exists in the primary healthcare setting and is rarely questioned by the responsible parties sitting upstream [65]. Gender inequality is considered as one of the key indicators in the primary healthcare setting that prevents effective decision-making for female DV victims [66]. Moreover, male dominance in the health sector is more likely to provide women with equal opportunities rather than equal rights, which can significantly impact victims or patients when they reveal their DV experiences [66]. However, male dominance and their hyper-masculine behaviour towards female victims compels victims to be male perpetrators' perpetual bait [64,66,67]. These changes should occur at the ecological level, and they must be addressed for the overall well-being of women.

Female patients who visit GPs with DV comorbidities have several concerns at the micro level. One concern is the GP's 'communication style'. DV victims have revealed communication as a common barrier preventing them from disclosing their DV experiences [5,34,51]. Australian studies have revealed that most victims would like to see some improvement in their GP's current communication style, which they claim is not conducive to feelings of trust and equality, inhibiting them from sharing their intimate life details [34,40]. Evidence demonstrates that mutually supportive communication supports victims to increase their self-confidence to discuss the topic with their GP [34,40]. This is a common desire among patients who use mental health services [47]. Many women who seek mental healthcare support report that they require their GPs to take a similar approach in terms of communication sensitivity in these spheres if they were to open up and share their stories [47]. Victims want to feel safe, which can only be achieved if the GP's communication style leads them to trust that this healthcare professional will not perceive them as being guilty for creating a situation that harmed their physical and mental health [68]. Primary healthcare providers require greater DV training and sensitive doctor–patient communication for these women to feel confident that the primary healthcare providers are competent in assisting them in their respective abusive situations [40].

Despite the reported competency gaps, the majority of healthcare professionals, including psychologists, psychiatrists and GPs, recognise DV as a serious health problem with huge social and economic costs to the country [7]. Proper training in sensitively screening victims will support healthcare professionals to identify DV victims [7]. However, this intention to improve skills and training in this area has not yet translated into a reduction in the skill gap of DV-based competence in primary healthcare professionals. Upskilling health practitioners should be considered as a given [7]. Nurses have reported feeling that they are not sufficiently aware of how DV works in terms of coercion and control, nor the inequities and power imbalances that drive and sustain it [69]. Insufficient skills and training to identify the signs of DV among healthcare professionals is reportedly common and covers the areas of communication skills, practical knowledge in DV, self-confidence, theoretical knowledge, skills to use relevant educational materials, proper knowledge of referral services, training in preparedness to face victims, skill development, identifying victims' behavioural patterns and accurate screening skills [7,34,41,69]. There is no current evidence demonstrating that sufficient training or resources are available for health staff to increase the skills and knowledge they need to gain the self-confidence and nuanced skills to identify DV safely in clinical settings [7,47,69–71].

Self-efficacy, self-confidence and self-esteem are reportedly key characteristics needed in primary healthcare professionals to work more effectively with DV victims and survivors [71]. Studies reveal that their perceived lack of self-efficacy (e.g., confident in being able to support victims and perpetrators in future nursing practices) is a main barrier preventing them from reaching out to potential sufferers and engaging in conversations with their patients about domestic abuse [71]. Low self-esteem in relation to these skills reportedly generates confusion and consequently unsuccessful assessments of their patients and low-quality reporting of cases [71]. Findings from the Australian context confirms that healthcare professionals are not confident in DV screening, identifying victims or referring victims to relevant support [7,69]. GPs' low confidence rates in their ability to properly and effectively assist their patients with DV combined with patient fear and low trust in GPs as people with whom they are likely to share their experiences, invariably results in faulty reports or incomplete assessments and low satisfaction for both GPs and patients [47]. For example, *"People (staff) are hesitant because they do not feel confident, they do not feel it is their job; they think that somebody else is better equipped to do it"* (P12, male, psychiatrist) [47]. The most common answers from nurses and midwives are the lack of privacy, knowledge, education and relevant resources [69]. Due to a lack of preparedness, nurses feel bad dealing with DV victims [71].

According to health professionals, they face numerous barriers when dealing with DV victims. Insufficient family violence patient resources, not having enough education resources, victims' uncertainty about their situation, lack of education and skill-based knowledge to deal with DV victims and not having specific training based on DV or family violence are most common critical issues [7].

Experts and scholars say that time is a crucial factor within the general practices. The duration of a GP consultation session is a decisive determinant in screening for family violence [7,68]. Studies reveals that 15 min of GP appointments are not sufficient to discuss DV experiences [7,22]. They suggest this issue is a sensitive concern [7]. During a general consultation is not the right time to discuss those experiences due to time barriers and heavy GP workloads [7]. The fact that GPs are unable to use this time to discuss DV experiences of their patients has been a significant issue for a long time [22,52]. There is considerable discussion on healthcare professionals' attitude, workloads, lack of training, inadequate consultation time, insufficient resource support and victims who present to the clinical health practices with their partners [52]. There is also an issue of health professionals' understanding their role: "Though I wanted to help victims, that is not my job" as one health professional described it [68]. These characteristics of general practices exist as barriers to identifying the signs of DV within the general practice setting.

Interventions and screening programs present as another area for improvement. Professionals have identified several improvements for implementing effective interventions in the primary healthcare setting [34,71]. For instance, DV interventions should address the victim's emotional needs [71]. Skill development should be compulsory to help practitioners identify the early symptoms DV within the primary healthcare setting [69]. Scholars present that most of the DV interventions are ineffective and do not provide the supporting environment to allow victims reveal personal experiences [68]. Almost all the nursing interventions concentrate on screening programs [68]. The healthcare system should find a more responsive service rather than screening [68]. Another issue that remains to be solved is the relationship between healthcare professional and the victim [68]. The tension between them leads healthcare workers to judge victims as abnormal and unacceptable [68]. For example, *"You, you talk to the patient, and you know, you get their story, "Oh, OK, yeah, you know that's terrible". Then, you talk to the psych services who know this patient very well and they give you the real story and it is completely different. You have been thrown off track by this patient"* (Sam) [68]. This kind of tension in the healthcare field needs to be solved to address the issue of DV [68]. To provide an effective response in primary healthcare services, it is imperative that professionals understand women's thinking and their experiences [68].

4. Discussion

This scoping review has located and discussed the most relevant articles on the reported barriers faced by Australian and New Zealand women experiencing DV in sharing their experiences with primary healthcare providers. Several journal articles, government organisations, non-government organisations and the Department of Health focus on the statistical data surroundings this serious public health concern [3,7,18–20,22–26,29,59]. The reason for this is that the incidence and prevalence of DV cases are gradually increasing—a fact that these responsible bodies are acutely aware of.

Within the primary healthcare settings and specifically in GP settings, it is a challenging task to identify DV victims unless they are willing to reveal their experiences of harassment, physical harm or sexual harm [10,54,56]. Victims are more likely to present with various other ill-health symptoms, such as sleep difficulties, mental health issues, injuries, fears or psychological factors that have been shown to be hidden and directly related to DV cases [5,10,34,39,42–45,48–50].

The review findings show that interventions implemented in the Australian primary healthcare and clinical settings to identify DV are not sufficient and are currently not operating in a way that achieves effective outcomes [5,32,34,38]. Additionally, DV screening programs are the most prominent intervention type within the Australian primary healthcare sector. Existing implementations are subject to several complications, including issues concerning self-completion surveys, self-reporting tools, selection bias in RCTs and not revealing the truth because of the fear of more intimate partner violence [5,10,32,34,36,38,56,59,60]. Despite the interventions, the majority of healthcare professionals are not aware of DV situations, victims, the signs or do not know how to react to the cases [10,34,47,51,68]. Healthcare professionals are in need of upskilling their knowledge, self-confidence, theoretical background, educational support and skill development regarding this social phenomenon.

Finally, gender imbalance and inequality between male and female health professionals within the primary healthcare setting appears to be a significant indicator of the quality of the health services provided within the primary healthcare settings and that offered by primary healthcare professionals [63–67]. Globally recognized strategies to reduce gender-based power differences at work, such as affirmative action, gender mainstreaming, gender equity training, and the encouraging of women into medicine degrees over nursing degrees is required to redress this imbalance in healthcare systems. This scoping review has identified that power imbalances exist not only in personal relationships between two human beings but also across medical relationships [66].

Limitations

There were a few limitations to this scoping review. To examine the topic, a broad range of journals and databases were searched. It was not the aim nor the intention to undertake a systematic literature review, and as such, the documents we located as a result of the search terms and syntax we employed did not yield a complete set of all possible articles on this topic. Future systematic reviews could specifically include a focus on words such as 'symptoms, comorbidities, detection, and interventions', for example. Search strategies were developed that reflected the immediate aims and objectives of the research, and provide a snapshot of what research is available to address a specific set of questions. However, the articles located were indeed able to provide the findings we needed to provide answers commensurate with the aims of this review. Moreover, the scoping review was limited to articles in the English language.

5. Conclusions

This scoping review collated the current evidence available within the scope of our search methodology on the many reasons that DV victims are reluctant to openly discuss their DV experience at the primary healthcare level. According to the perspective of Public Health, primary healthcare professionals play a vital role in preventing and managing DV against women, however, this is currently undermined due to a range of barriers to communicating situations and symptoms to clinicians in private settings A core finding emerging from the review was that the current power imbalance between male and female staff across allied and clinical health sectors be remedied. This issue has become a staple problem in the social structures and health settings throughout the decades and is particularly sensitive in the realm of DV detection and interventions. Moreover, this power imbalance is considered as a general and normal occurrence within the Australian primary healthcare setting, which is highly problematic. It is of concern that this power imbalance seeps into any social structures, given that these women already face massive power imbalances in their day-to-day lives.

The review also concluded that while screening is the principal intervention tool used to identify DV victims within GP centres and other primary healthcare service providers, it is not always confidently applied by practitioners nor sought out by DV victims during visits. Innovative interventions are needed within these settings, such as effective and more nuanced, or sensitive DV screening tools, risk assessments and case study findings to generate ways in which a rapport between GP and patient can be generated and protected during screenings. Accurate, sensitive, and safe screening can support health providers to identify victims at the right time [12]. GPs also need to become far more educated regarding the clusters of comorbidities that typically accompany a DV victims health report. While the DV itself may not be communicated in clinical settings, all healthcare providers need to be educated on the 'red flags' such as sleep problems, anxiety, and substance use that often point to an underlying set of DV conditions. On the other hand, victims need to be made much more aware of benefits of screening programs and other DV prevention tools. Victims are often not aware of what support is available for them and primary healthcare providers often fail to refer victims to such support.

Further research is needed to collect more accurate and reliable data regarding disclosure in healthcare settings. Specifically, there is a concerning deficiency in population-based studies and research, which could be the most effective for researchers, scholars, public health practitioners, policy advocates and primary healthcare service providers. Health policymakers must be aware of equal rights with equal opportunities for female workers in the primary healthcare setting. Policymakers must also pay attention to public health norms, due to the importance of women's overall health consequently reflecting the health of the country's future generations. Advocating for changing the social structure is of the utmost importance to ensure both male and female professionals are present at the first layer of Australian healthcare. This should be considered as a mandatory requirement to empower women.

Author Contributions: J.C.R.: Wrote the original draft and conceptualized the paper; J.C.R., N.M.P., J.-A.C. and J.K.: Contributed to methodology, analysis, writing—review, and editing; J.-A.C.: Supervised the team. All authors have read and agreed to the published version of the manuscript.

Funding: This research received no external funding.

Institutional Review Board Statement: Not applicable.

Informed Consent Statement: Not applicable.

Data Availability Statement: Not applicable.

Conflicts of Interest: The authors declare no conflict of interest.

References

1. International Committee of the Red Cross. Addressing Sexual Violence. 2020. Available online: https://www.icrc.org/en/what-we-do/sexual-violence (accessed on 21 April 2021).
2. United Nations. What is Domestic Abuse? 2020. Available online: https://www.un.org/en/coronavirus/what-is-domestic-abuse (accessed on 21 April 2021).
3. Rees, S.; Silove, D.; Chey, T.; Ivancic, L.; Steel, Z.; Creamer, M.; Teeson, M.; Bryant, R.; McFarlane, A.C.; Mills, K.L.; et al. Lifetime prevalence of gender-based violence in women and the relationship with mental disorders and psychosocial function. *Am. Med. Assoc.* **2011**, *306*, 513–521. [CrossRef]
4. Wendt, S. *Domestic Violence in Rural Australia*; Federation Press: Annandale, Australia, 2009.

5. Hegarty, K.; O'Doherty, L.; Taft, A.; Chondros, P.; Brown, S.; Valpied, J.; Astbury, J.; Taket, A.; Gold, L.; Feder, G.; et al. Screening and counseling in the primary care setting for women who have experienced intimate partner violence (WEAVE): A cluster randomized trial. *Lancet* **2013**, *382*, 249–258. [CrossRef] [PubMed]
6. United Nations. *Taking Stock of the Global Partnership for Development*; United Nations: New York, NY, USA, 2015. Available online: https://www.un.org/millenniumgoals/pdf/MDG_Gap_2015_E_web.pdf (accessed on 21 April 2021).
7. Soh, H.J.; Grigg, J.; Gurvich, C.; Gavrilidis, E.; Kulkarni, J. Family violence: An insight into perspectives and practices of Australian health practitioners. *J. Interpers. Violence* **2018**, *36*, NP2391–NP2409. [CrossRef] [PubMed]
8. World Health Organisation. Violence against Women. 2020. Available online: https://www.who.int/news-room/fact-sheets/detail/violence-against-women (accessed on 25 April 2021).
9. Garcia-Moreno, C.; Watts, C. Violence against women: An urgent public health priority. *Bull. World Health Organ.* **2011**, *89*, 2. [CrossRef] [PubMed]
10. Hegarty, K.L.; O'Doherty, L.J.; Chondros, P.; Valpied, J.; Taft, A.J.; Astbury, J.; Gunn, J.M. Effect of type and severity of intimate partner violence on women's health and service use: Findings from a primary care trial of women afraid of their partners. *J. Interpers. Violence* **2013**, *28*, 273–294. [CrossRef]
11. Szalacha, L.A.; Hughes, T.L.; McNair, R.; Loxton, D. Mental health, sexual identity, and interpersonal violence: Findings from the Australian longitudinal women's health study. *BMC Women's Health* **2017**, *17*, 94. [CrossRef]
12. Fiolet, S. Intimate partner violence: Australian nurses and midwives trained to provide care? *Aust. Nurs. J.* **2013**, *20*, 37. [PubMed]
13. U.S. Department of Health & Human Services. Effects of Violence against Women. 2019. Available online: https://www.womenshealth.gov/relationships-and-safety/effects-violence-against-women (accessed on 1 May 2021).
14. Carton, H.; Egan, V. The dark triad and intimate partner violence. *Personal. Individ. Differ.* **2017**, *105*, 84–88. [CrossRef]
15. House, A.A. Intimate partner violence. *Can. Med. Assoc. J.* **2015**, *187*, 1312. [CrossRef]
16. Taket, A.; O'Doherty, L.; Valpied, J.; Hegarty, K. What do Australian women experiencing intimate partner abuse want from family and friends? *Qual. Health Res.* **2016**, *24*, 983–996. [CrossRef]
17. Dillon, G.; Hussain, R.; Kibele, E.; Rahman, O.; Loxton, D. Influence of intimate partner violence on domestic relocation in Metropolitan and Non-Metropolitan young Australian Women. *Violence Against Women* **2016**, *22*, 1597–1620. [CrossRef] [PubMed]
18. Mission Australia. Domestic and Family Violence Statistics. 2020. Available online: https://www.missionaustralia.com.au/domestic-and-family-violence-statistics (accessed on 3 May 2021).
19. Australian Institute of Health and Welfare. Family, Domestic and Sexual Violence. 2019. Available online: https://www.aihw.gov.au/reports-data/behaviours-risk-factors/domestic-violence/overview (accessed on 5 May 2021).
20. Puccetti, M.; Greville, H.; Robinson, M.; White, D.; Papertalk, L.; Thompson, S.C. Exploring readiness fir change: Knowledge and attitude towards family violence among community members and service providers engaged in primary prevention in regional Australia. *Int. J. Environ. Res. Public Health* **2019**, *16*, 4215. [CrossRef] [PubMed]
21. Australian Bureau of Statistics. Personal Safety, Australia-Statistic for Family, Domestic, Sexual Violence, Physical Assault, Partner Emotional Abuse, Child Abuse, Sexual Harassment, Stalking and Safety. 2017. Available online: https://www.abs.gov.au/statistics/people/crime-and-justice/personal-safety-australia/latest-release#about-the-personal-safety-survey (accessed on 6 May 2021).
22. Meuleners, L.B.; Lee, A.H.; Xia, J.; Fraser, M.; Hendrie, D. Interpersonal violence presentation to general practitioners in Western Australia: Implications for rural and community health. *Aust. Health Rev.* **2011**, *35*, 70–74. [CrossRef] [PubMed]
23. Hooker, L.; Versteegh, L.; Lindgren, H.; Taft, A. Differences in help-seeking behaviours and perceived helpfulness of services between abused and non-abused women: A cross-sectional survey of Australian postpartum women. *Health Soc. Care Community* **2019**, *28*, 958–968. [CrossRef]
24. Gartland, D.; Woolhouse, H.; Mensah, F.K.; Hegarty, K.; Hiscook, H.; Brown, S.J. The case for early intervention to reduce the impact of intimate partner abuse on child outcomes: Results of an Australian cohort of first-time mothers. *Birth* **2014**, *41*, 374–383. [CrossRef] [PubMed]
25. Australian Bureau of Statistics. Recoded Crime—Victims, Australia. 2019. Available online: https://www.abs.gov.au/statistics/people/crime-and-justice/recorded-crime-victims-australia/latest-release (accessed on 6 May 2021).
26. McGarry, A. Older women, intimate partner violence and mental health: A consideration of the particular issue for health and healthcare practice. *J. Clin. Nurs.* **2017**, *26*, 2177–2191. [CrossRef] [PubMed]
27. Peterman, A. *Pandemics and Violence against Women and Children*; Centre for Global Development: Washington, DC, USA, 2020.
28. van Gelder, N.E.; van Haalen, D.L.; Ekker, K.; Ligthart, S.A.; Oertelt-Prigione, S. Professionals' views on working in the field of domestic violence and abuse during the first wave of COVID-19: A qualitative study in the Netherlands. *BMC Health Serv. Res.* **2021**, *21*, 624. [CrossRef]
29. Crombie, N.; Hooker, L.; Resenhofer, S. Nurse and midwifery education and intimate partner violence: A scoping review. *J. Clin. Nurs.* **2017**, *26*, 2100–2125. [CrossRef]
30. Tower, M.; Rowe, J.; Wallis, M. Normalizing policies of inaction—The case of health care in Australia for women affected by domestic violence. *Health Care Women Int.* **2011**, *32*, 855–868. [CrossRef]
31. Murray, S.; Powell, A. "What's the problem?" Australian public policy constructions of domestic and family violence. *Violence Against Women* **2009**, *15*, 532–552. [CrossRef]

32. Taft, A.J.; Hooker, L.; Humphreys, C.; Hegarty, K.; Walter, R.; Adams, C. Maternal and child health nurse screening and care for mothers experiencing domestic violence (MOVE): A cluster randomized control trial. *BMC Med.* **2015**, *13*, 150. [CrossRef] [PubMed]
33. Signorelli, M.C.; Taft, A.; Pereira, P.P.G. Intimate partner violence against women and healthcare in Australia: Charting the scene. *Cienc. Saude Coletivia* **2012**, *17*, 1037–1048. [CrossRef] [PubMed]
34. O'Doherty, L.; Taket, A.; Valpied, J.; Hegarty, K. Receiving care for intimate partner violence in primary care: Barriers and enablers for women participating in the weave randomised controlled trial. *Soc. Sci. Med.* **2016**, *160*, 35–42. [CrossRef] [PubMed]
35. Hegarty, L. The GP's Role in Assisting Family Violence Victims. 2019. Available online: https://www.ausdoc.com.au/therapy-update/gps-role-assisting-family-violence-victims (accessed on 10 May 2021).
36. Spangaro, J.M.; Zwi, A.B.; Poulos, R.G.; Man, W.Y.N. Who tells and what happens: Disclosure and health service responses to screening for intimate partner violence. *Health Soc. Care Community* **2010**, *18*, 671–680. [CrossRef]
37. Mertin, P.; Moyle, S.; Veremeenko, K. Intimate partner violence and women's presentation in general practice settings: Barriers to disclosure and implications for therapeutic interventions. *Clin. Psychol.* **2014**, *19*, 140–146. [CrossRef]
38. Hegarty, K.L.; Gunn, J.M.; O'Doherty, L.J.; Taft, A.; Chondros, P.; Feder, G.; Astbury, J.; Brown, S. Women's evaluation of abuse and violence care in general practice: A cluster randomized controlled trial (weave). *BMC Public Health* **2010**, *10*, 2. [CrossRef]
39. Francis, L.; Loxton, D.; James, C. The culture of pretence: A hidden barrier to recognizing, disclosing and ending domestic violence. *J. Clin. Nurs.* **2016**, *26*, 2202–2214. [CrossRef]
40. Hegarty, K.L.; O'Doherty, L.J.; Astbury, J.; Gunn, J. Identifying intimate partner violence when screening for health and lifestyle issues among women attending general practice. *Aust. J. Prim. Health* **2012**, *18*, 327–331. [CrossRef]
41. Hegarty, K.L.; Bush, R. Prevalence and associations of partner abuse in women attending general practice: A cross-sectional survey. *Aust. N. Z. J. Public Health* **2002**, *26*, 437–442. [CrossRef]
42. Astbury, J.; Bruck, D.; Loxton, D. Forced sex: A critical factor in the sleep difficulties of young Australian women. *Violence Vict.* **2011**, *26*, 53–72. [CrossRef]
43. Bruck, D.; Astbury, J. Population study on the predictors of sleeping difficulties in young Australian women. *Behav. Sleep Med.* **2012**, *10*, 84–95. [CrossRef] [PubMed]
44. Mertin, P.; Mohr, P.B. Incidence and correlates of posttraumatic stress disorders in Australian victims of domestic violence. *J. Fam. Violence* **2000**, *15*, 411–422. [CrossRef]
45. Stam, M.T.; Ford-Gilboe, M.; Regan, S. Primary health care service use among women who have recently left an abusive partner: Income and racialization, unmet need, fits of services, and health. *Health Care Women Int.* **2015**, *36*, 161–187. [CrossRef] [PubMed]
46. Campbell, J.C. Health consequences of intimate partner violence. *Lancet* **2002**, *359*, 1331–1336. [CrossRef]
47. Rose, D.; Kylee, T.; Woodall, A.; Morgan, C.; Feder, G.; Howard, L. Barriers and facilitators of disclosures of domestic violence by mental health service users: A qualitative study. *Br. J. Psychiatry* **2011**, *198*, 189–194. [CrossRef]
48. Sharman, L.S.; Douglas, H.; Price, E.; Sheeran, N.; Dingle, G. Associations between unintended pregnancy, domestic violence and sexual assault in a population of Queensland women. *Psychiatry Psychol. Law* **2018**, *26*, 541–552. [CrossRef]
49. Taft, A.; Watson, L. Depression and termination of pregnancy (induced abortion) in a national cohort of young Australian women: The confounding effect of women's experience of violence. *BMC Public Health* **2008**, *8*, 75. [CrossRef]
50. Martin-de-las-Heras, S.; Velasco, C.; Luna, J.; Martin, A. Unintended pregnancy and intimate partner violence around pregnancy in a population-based study. *J. Aust. Coll. Midwives* **2015**, *28*, 101–105. [CrossRef]
51. Moynihan, R.N. Domestic violence: Can doctors do more to help? *Med. J. Aust.* **2012**, *197*, 75. [CrossRef]
52. Taft, A.J.; Small, R.; Humphreys, C.; Hegarty, K.; Walter, R.; Adams, C.; Agis, P. Enhanced maternal and child health nurse care for women experiencing intimate partner/family violence: Protocol for MOVE, a cluster randomized trial of screening and referral in primary health care. *BMC Public Health* **2012**, *12*, 811. [CrossRef]
53. Rabin, R.F.; Jennings, J.M.; Campbell, J.C.; Bair-Merritt, M.H. Intimate partner violence screening tools; A systematic review. *American journal of preventive medicine*. **2009**, *36*, 439–445.e4. [CrossRef] [PubMed]
54. O'Doherty, L.; Hegarty, K.; Ramsey, J.; Davidson, L.; Feder, G.; Taft, A. Screening women for intimate partner violence in healthcare settings. *Cochrane Database Syst. Rev.* **2015**, CD007007. [CrossRef] [PubMed]
55. Commonwealth of Australia. *Screening, Risk Assessment and Safety Planning*; Commonwealth of Australia: Barton, Australia, 2010. Available online: https://www.avertfamilyviolence.com.au/wp-content/uploads/sites/4/2013/06/Screening_Risk_Assessment.pdf (accessed on 15 June 2021).
56. MacMillan, H.L.; Wathen, N.; Jamieson, E.; Boyle, M.H.; Shannon, H.S.; Ford-Gilboe, M.; Worster, A.; Lent, B.; Coben, J.H.; Campbell, J.C.; et al. Screening for intimate partner violence in healthcare setting: A randomized control trial. *JAMA* **2009**, *302*, 493–501. [CrossRef] [PubMed]
57. Johns Hopkins Medicine. Routine Screening. 2021. Available online: https://www.hopkinsmedicine.org/health/treatment-tests-and-therapies/routine-screenings (accessed on 15 June 2021).
58. The University of Queensland. Domestic Violence Case Studies. 2018. Available online: https://law.uq.edu.au/research/dv/using-law-leaving-domestic-violence/case-studies (accessed on 15 June 2021).
59. Parkinson, D. Investigating the increase in domestic violence post disaster: An Australian case study. *J. Interpers. Violence* **2017**, *34*, 2333–2362. [CrossRef]

60. McLaughlin, H.; Robbins, R.; Bellamy, C.; Banks, C.; Thackray, D. Adult social work and high-risk domestic violence cases. *J. Soc. Work* **2018**, *18*, 288–306. [CrossRef]
61. Spangaro, J.M.; Poulos, R.; Zwi, A. Pandora doesn't live here anymore: Normalization of screening for intimate partner violence in Australian antenatal, mental health, and substance abuse services. *Violence Vict.* **2011**, *26*, 130–144. [CrossRef]
62. Rosenman, R.; Tennekoon, V.; Hill, L.G. Measuring bias in self-reporting. *Int. J. Behav. Healthc. Res.* **2011**, *2*, 320–332. [CrossRef]
63. Davies, S.E. Gender empowerment in the health aid sector: Locating best practice in the Australian context. *Aust. J. Int. Aff.* **2018**, *72*, 520–534. [CrossRef]
64. Anderson, K.L.; Umberson, D. Gendering Violence: Masculinity and power in men's accounts of domestic violence. *Gend. Soc.* **2001**, *15*, 358–380. [CrossRef]
65. Ollivier, R.; Aston, M.; Price, S. Let's talk about sex: A feminist poststructural approach to addressing sexual health in the healthcare setting. *J. Clin. Nurs.* **2018**, *28*, 695–702. [CrossRef]
66. Kuskoff, E.; Parsell, C. Preventing domestic violence by changing Australian gender relations: Issues and considerations. *Aust. Soc. Work* **2019**, *73*, 227–235. [CrossRef]
67. Berns, N. Degendering the problem and gendering the blame: Political discourse on women and violence. *Gend. Soc.* **2001**, *15*, 262–281. [CrossRef]
68. Tower, M.; Rowe, J.; Wallis, M. Reconceptualising health and health care for women affected by domestic violence. *Contemp. Nurse* **2012**, *42*, 216–225. [CrossRef]
69. Hooker, L.; Bernadette, W.; Verrinder, G. Domestic violence screening in maternal and child health nursing practice: A scoping review. *Contemp. Nurse* **2012**, *42*, 198–215. [CrossRef] [PubMed]
70. Cleak, H.; Hunt, G.; Hardy, F.; Brett, D.; Bell, J. Health staff responses to domestic and family violence: The case for training to build confidence and skills. *Aust. Soc. Work* **2020**, *74*, 42–54. [CrossRef]
71. Beccaria, G.; Beccaria, L.; Dawson, R.; Gorman, D.; Harris, J.A.; Hossain, D. Nursing student's perception and understanding of intimate partner violence. *Nurse Educ. Today* **2013**, *33*, 907–911. [CrossRef] [PubMed]

Disclaimer/Publisher's Note: The statements, opinions and data contained in all publications are solely those of the individual author(s) and contributor(s) and not of MDPI and/or the editor(s). MDPI and/or the editor(s) disclaim responsibility for any injury to people or property resulting from any ideas, methods, instructions or products referred to in the content.

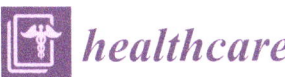

Article

The Impact of Sexual Violence on Quality of Life and Mental Wellbeing in Transgender and Gender-Diverse Adolescents and Young Adults: A Mixed-Methods Approach

Aisa Burgwal [1,*], Jara Van Wiele [1] and Joz Motmans [2]

1. Transgender Infopunt, Ghent University Hospital, Corneel Heymanslaan 10, 9000 Ghent, Belgium; jaravanwiele@hotmail.com
2. Center for Sexology and Gender, Ghent University Hospital, Corneel Heymanslaan 10, 9000 Ghent, Belgium; joz.motmans@uzgent.be
* Correspondence: a.burgwal@amsterdamumc.nl

Abstract: Transgender (trans) and gender-diverse (GD) adolescents and young adults have remained largely invisible in health research. Previous research shows worse outcomes in health indicators for trans and GD people, compared to cisgender controls. Research on the impact of sexual violence focuses on mainly cisgender female adult victims. This study assessed the impact of sexual violence on the quality of life (QoL) and mental wellbeing (GHQ-12) among trans and GD adolescents and young adults, while taking into account the possible role of gender nonconformity in sexual violence and mental wellbeing. An online, anonymous survey and interviews/focus groups were conducted between October 2021 and May 2022 in Belgium. Multiple analyses of covariance (ANCOVAs) were used to assess the associations between sexual violence, mental wellbeing, and gender nonconformity, while controlling for different background variables (gender identity, sexual orientation, age, economic vulnerability, etc.). The interviews and focus groups were used to validate associations between variables that were hypothesized as important. The quantitative sample consisted of 110 respondents between 15 and 25 years old, with 30 trans respondents (27.3%) and 80 GD respondents (72.7%). A total of 73.6% reported experiences with sexual violence over the past two years ($n = 81$). The mean QoL score was 5.3/10, and the mean GHQ-12 score was 6.6/12. Sexual violence was not significantly associated with QoL ($p = 0.157$) and only marginally significantly associated with GHQ-12 ($p = 0.05$). Changing one's physical appearance to conform to gender norms, out of fear of getting attacked, discriminated against, or harassed was significantly associated with QoL ($p = 0.009$) and GHQ-12 ($p = 0.041$). The association between sexual violence and changing one's physical appearance to conform to gender norms was analyzed, to assess a possible mediation effect of sexual violence on mental wellbeing. No significant association was found ($p = 0.261$). However, the interviews suggest that sexual violence is associated with changing one's physical appearance, but this association is not limited to only trans and GD victims of sexual violence. Non-victims also adjust their appearance, out of fear of future sexual victimization. Together with the high proportion of sexual violence, as well as the lower average QoL and higher average GHQ-12 scores among trans and GD adolescents and young adults, compared to general population statistics, this highlights the need for policy makers to create more inclusive environments.

Keywords: transgender; gender-diverse; sexual violence; gender expression; avoidance behavior; quality of life; GHQ-12

Citation: Burgwal, A.; Van Wiele, J.; Motmans, J. The Impact of Sexual Violence on Quality of Life and Mental Wellbeing in Transgender and Gender-Diverse Adolescents and Young Adults: A Mixed-Methods Approach. *Healthcare* **2023**, *11*, 2281. https://doi.org/10.3390/healthcare11162281

Academic Editor: Juan Carlos Sierra

Received: 11 July 2023
Revised: 27 July 2023
Accepted: 8 August 2023
Published: 13 August 2023

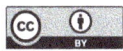

Copyright: © 2023 by the authors. Licensee MDPI, Basel, Switzerland. This article is an open access article distributed under the terms and conditions of the Creative Commons Attribution (CC BY) license (https://creativecommons.org/licenses/by/4.0/).

1. Introduction

Media coverage in recent years shows that incidents of sexual violence against transgender (trans) and gender-diverse (GD) adolescents and young adults remain a reality. At the same time, a large proportion of trans and GD individuals do not officially report sexual violence [1,2]. The visibility of various gender expressions and identities has increased as well. On the one hand, this increased social and political visibility raises the chance of coming into contact with trans and GD individuals, which in turn has a positive effect on attitudes towards this group [3–6]. On the other hand, there may also be social and personal disadvantages associated with an increased visibility. As trans and GD people become more visible, and feel more comfortable being open about their gender identity, they are also more likely to become victims to negative reactions and even violence [7–11].

Consistent with the Standards of Care 8, we use the term transgender and gender-diverse (trans and GD) to be as broad and inclusive as possible, when describing members of the many diverse communities of people with gender identities or expressions that differ from their sex assigned at birth. The term was chosen with the intention of being as inclusive as possible, and to highlight the many diverse gender identities and expressions among trans and GD people [12].

1.1. Mental WellBeing of Trans and Gender-Diverse Individuals

The social impact on a person because of their belonging to a minority group related to sex and/or gender may lead to minority stress [13,14]. The minority stress model suggests that poor physical and/or mental health among sexual minorities can, to a large extent, be explained by stress factors caused by a hostile les-, homo-, and bi- (LGB)phobic culture, often resulting in persistent bullying, discrimination, and victimization [14–16]. While the minority stress model was developed with regard to LGB people, research has shown that trans and GD people suffer from gender minority stressors too [17–22].

The current study assesses quality of life (QoL) and mental wellbeing (GHQ-12). Various studies show that minority groups, such as trans and GD individuals, score lower on mental wellbeing outcomes than the general population [2,23–28]. A few studies have assessed wellbeing within this group, though not solely in a Belgian context, or solely among trans and GD adolescents and young adults. The EU LGBTI II study assessed QoL among European trans and GD adolescents and young adults aged 15–24, where a mean QoL score of 5.2/10 was found, which was significantly lower than that among the QoL of trans and GD respondents aged 25 and older, for whom a mean of 6.1/10 was found ($p < 0.001$) [25]. The score was also lower than the average of 7.6/10 among the general Belgian population aged 18 to 24, measured using the European Quality of Life Survey [26]. General mental wellbeing can be measured using the General Health Questionnaire 12 (GHQ-12, short version). This scale has been validated within the general Dutch-speaking population, where an average Cronbach's alpha of 0.90 was detected. The scale has also been validated within the Flemish transgender population, where a high Cronbach's alpha ($\alpha = 0.91$) was found. The Flemish study of Motmans, T'Sjoen and Meier [2] assessed the GHQ-12 score among trans people, regardless of age. The mean GHQ-12 score was 3.9/12, and was significantly higher ($p < 0.001$) than the Belgian mean score of 1.3/12 [27]. Other studies find similar results when the GHQ-12 scores of trans and GD individuals are compared to those of cisgender individuals [23,24,28].

1.2. Sexual Violence

The proportional rates of sexual violence among trans and GD adolescents and young adults vary considerably, ranging from 31.7% to 42.0% [2,29]. This variability is largely due to differences in the conceptual and operational definitions of sexual violence, which limit the comparability of existing studies, and the ability to draw conclusions [30,31]. Age also seems to be of importance when assessing sexual violence. Various studies highlight the association between sexual violence and age, with younger people reporting more sexual violence [25,32]. Focusing on Belgium, where the current study was conducted, only one nationally representative study is available that assessed sexual violence among LGBTI+ people [32]. This study found that 68% of the LGBTI+ respondents were confronted with at least one type of sexual victimization in the last year. To allow a comparison with the results of the current study with the study of Keygnaert, De Schrijver, Cismaru Inescu, Schapansky, Nobels, Hahaut, Stappers, De Bauw, Lemonne, Renard, Weewauters,

Nisen, Vander Beken and Vandeviver [32], the same definition of sexual violence was used, following the definition provided by the World Health Organization [33] (WHO). The WHO suggests a broad definition of sexual violence, including hands-off and hands-on behaviors, and does not specify the gender of the victim or the perpetrator. Hands-off sexual violence refers to violence without any physical contact between the perpetrator and the victim (e.g., verbal or visual sexual harassment). This type of sexual violence can take place online and offline. Hands-on sexual violence refers to violence where physical contact between the perpetrator and victim is present (e.g., sexual abuse with/without penetration, (attempted) rape).

The current study will focus on sexual violence and its associated factors in the Flemish general trans and GD population aged 15 to 25. By relying on the WHO definition of sexual violence, well-established, existing measures are used to incorporate the proportions of sexual violence, and to avoid a gender bias in the item wording.

1.3. Impact of Sexual Violence

The Minority Stress Model by Meyer [13,14] emphasizes that individuals belonging to a minority group face additional stressors that impact their wellbeing. Effective experiences with violence, as well as awareness of existing stigma, cause someone to experience minority stress. The most external and explicit sources of minority stress that trans and GD people can experience are actual experiences with violence (including sexual violence).

The impact of violence on physical and mental health depends on the type of violence, the frequency, the characteristics of the perpetrator, and the characteristics of the victim [8]. Motmans, T'Sjoen and Meier [2] showed that experiencing sexual violence was associated with significantly lower psychological wellbeing (GHQ-12) ($p = 0.007$). The EU Agency for Fundamental Rights [29] also found that trans and GD respondents who indicated that they had experienced sexual or physical violence in the past five years showed a significantly lower satisfaction with life than non-victims ($p < 0.001$). This difference remained significant when only 15–24 year old trans and GD victims of sexual or physical violence were compared with non-victims ($p < 0.001$).

Violence specifically aimed at the minority status of the individual (hate crime) causes an increase in feelings of insecurity and hypervigilance [11,34–37]. Walters, et al. [38] found that trans and GD people are even more likely to have increased levels of vigilance, vulnerability, and anxiety compared to cisgender LGB people. Moreover, individuals who experience a transphobic incident are more aware of their own stigmatized status than those who have not experienced violence.

1.4. Motives for Sexual Violence

There are a number of theories about the motives for committing anti-LGBT+ violence, which also applies to transphobic violence. One of the assumed motives underlying anti-LGBT+ violence is gender nonconformity.

Gender Nonconformity

Gender nonconformity is a broad term referring to people who do not behave in a way that conforms to the traditional expectations of their gender, or whose gender expression does not fit neatly into a category [39]. Stigma based on gender identity/expression works in a way wherein only two gender options are considered valid in our society: male and female. All gender options other than male and female are devalued [40,41]. A cisgender identity is as a result ideologically equated with 'normal' masculinity and femininity, while a transgender or gender-diverse identity is equated with a transgression of these gender norms [42–45]. Several studies show that transphobic violence stems from an irrational fear of those who do not conform to cultural gender norms, rather than from being provoked by the minority status of the victim themself [40,41]. For trans and GD individuals, a person may not know whether an individual lives fully in a different gender role, or has undergone gender reassignment treatment. However, trans and GD victims of public violence are often those who are visibly trans or GD people (those individuals who cannot be categorized into a clear male or female categorization, or those who still show clear characteristics of their sex assigned at birth) [2]. Behaving or dressing in a way that, according to social norms, only fits the opposite gender, or does not fit into one of the binary gender roles, increases the chance of violent reactions [7,25,46]. This assumes that those who do not exceed gender norms are less likely to experience violence [7,45]. In addition, a study conducted among people who did not belong to a sexual or gender minority group showed that the perception of a non-heterosexual orientation or a transgender identity also led to violence. This confirms the theory that it is not the trans or GD identity itself that predicts the degree of violence, but rather the degree of gender nonconformity [47]. As a result, violence due to gender nonconformity can lead to trans and GD people adjusting their own behavior in order to avoid being in violent situations again [2,36]. Motmans, T'Sjoen and Meier [2] showed that experiencing a sexual transphobic incident caused 40.4% to avoid certain places/people. The study by the EU Agency for Fundamental Rights [29] also showed that 23.4% of trans and GD respondents often-to-always adjusted their appearance out of fear of getting attacked, threatened, or discriminated against. A significant association was found between sexual/physical violence and physical appearance modification. Trans respondents who reported experiences of sexual or physical violence in the past five years significantly more often changed their appearance, out of fear of becoming a victim (again) ($p < 0.001$).

1.5. Research Goals

Various studies have assessed the association between sexual violence and mental wellbeing outcomes [2,25,32,48], and between sexual violence and gender nonconformity [25,42,46,49] among trans and GD people. This article assesses the association between sexual violence and quality of life/mental wellbeing among trans and GD adolescents and young adults (15–25 years of age), and examines the role of gender nonconformity in each of these variables. Based on the literature, it is hypothesized that sexual violence is significantly associated with lower mental health outcomes, even when different sociodemographic background variables are taken into account. Avoidance behavior, especially changing one's physical appearance out of fear of being attacked, discriminated against, or harassed, will also be taken into account, when assessing wellbeing. This type of behavior is associated with gender nonconformity, as changing one's appearance often refers to a greater degree of gender conformity. It is hypothesized that changing one's physical appearance will also be significantly associated with both a lower quality of life, and lower mental wellbeing. There is emerging evidence that, in some situations, tests of mediated effects can be statistically significant when the direct effect of the independent variable (e.g., sexual violence) on the outcome variable (e.g., mental wellbeing) is not statistically significant [50–52]. If no direct association between sexual violence and mental wellbeing is found, then an indirect mediation effect through changing one's physical appearance is expected, suggesting full mediation. In comparison with non-victims, it is hypothesized that sexual violence victims will change their physical appearance significantly more often to be more gender conforming, which leads to a significantly lower mental wellbeing.

2. Materials and Methods

This study was conducted through the Ghent University Hospital (UZ Ghent), and was funded by the Flemish Government. In 2020, the Equal Opportunities Service proposed to study the experiences with violence of LGBTI+ people, in order to gather empirical evidence about the experiences of LGBTI+ people across Belgium that could be used to improve policy-making and work with LGBTI+ communities. The current article focuses on trans and GD youth with a range of identities, including trans girls (i.e., individuals assigned male at birth, who identify as female or another feminine identity), trans boys (i.e., individuals assigned female at birth, who identify as male or another masculine identity), and gender-diverse or non-binary youth (i.e., individuals who identify as neither male or female, as both male and female, or as another gender identity that is not congruent with their sex assigned at birth).

2.1. Study Design

The results in this article were obtained using a cross-sectional, mixed-method design. Experiences of violence were assessed retrospectively, using an online survey, and in-person interviews/focus groups. The respondents who left their contact details at the end of the survey were followed up for an interview, or for participation in a focus group. The main study focused on the experiences with violence of the entire LGBTI+ group. The current article only focuses on the 15–25 year old trans and GD respondents who participated in the main study.

2.2. Data Collection Method

The research has been approved by the Commission for Medical Ethics of the Ghent University Hospital. Participants were recruited through the online survey in the study "Genoeg–Enough–Assez". The survey was hosted by the online survey platform RedCap, and was accessible between October 2021 and January 2022. The interviews and focus groups were conducted between February 2022 and May 2022. LGBTI+ people aged 15 years or older who had lived in Belgium for the past two years were invited to complete an anonymous survey. A convenience sampling strategy was applied, through which the online survey was promoted via posters, flyers, and online (social media). Participants were recruited at different LGBTI+ and non-LGBTI+ events, such as Belgian prides, parties, in queer cafés, during slam poetry events, etc. The LGBTI+ organizations involved in the study helped to reach out to respondents. After each month of data collection, a preliminary analysis was conducted, to check for representativeness, in comparison to the general Belgian population statistics. Based on the results, extra recruitment occasions were scheduled that were specifically aimed at recruiting older LGBTI+ respondents, respondents with a minority ethnic–cultural background, and intersex respondents. At the end of the online survey, people had the option to leave their contact details if they wished to be invited to an interview/focus group. Anyone identifying with an LGBTI+ label could participate, regardless of whether they had experience with violence.

The current article only focuses on the trans and GD respondents who are living in the Flemish/Brussels Capital Region of Belgium, and who are between 15 and 25 years of age. Participants older than 25 years of age, living in the Walloon Region, or with a cisgender identity, were excluded from the analysis. Participants from the Walloon Region were excluded due to there being too small a sample size ($n = 5$). Those who did not sign the informed consent, or who ended the survey before the start of the questions about experiences with violence, were also excluded from the analysis. Of the 110 respondents that fell within the above-defined group and participated in the survey, 32 respondents left their contact details at the end of the survey. All these respondents were invited to participate in the follow-up qualitative part of the study. An invitation to an interview, or an invitation to participate in a focus group, was predetermined at random. In the end, five respondents agreed to participate, of which four were interviewed, and one participated in a focus group.

As the main study focused on LGBTI+ people in general, the focus group also included four cisgender LGB people. Their data were excluded from the qualitative analyses. For both the survey and the interviews/focus group, informed consent forms were signed. It took on average 30 min to complete the survey, and the interviews took approximately one hour, and were audio-recorded. Participants received a debriefing after the survey and interview/focus group, with the contact information of resources that they could reach out to after participating in the study. Participants did not receive an incentive to participate.

2.3. Data Analysis Method

Data analysis of the quantitative survey was performed using SPSS for Windows, v28 [53]. A power analysis was conducted to determine the number of participants in this study [54–57]. Both quality of life and mental wellbeing were continuous variables, and the errors of both dependent variables did not deviate from normality. A series of univariate analyses (ANCOVAs) were performed, to test the hypothesis of a significant difference in mental wellbeing outcomes between young trans and GD individuals who had experienced SV and those who had not, while controlling for different socio-demographic control variables (sexual orientation, sex assigned at birth, gender identity, region, educational level, work situation, relationship status, ethnic–cultural minority, religious minority, minority due to disability status, age, economic vulnerability, and avoidance behaviors). Avoidance behaviors consist of hiding one's sexual orientation (for example, not holding hands with a romantic partner in public), and changing one's appearance, out of fear of being attacked, discriminated against, or harassed. Age, economic vulnerability, and both of the avoidance behaviors were used as continuous control variables during the analyses. A p value of <0.05 was considered to be statistically significant. The p-value is only reported when the control variable is significantly associated with the outcome variable. To achieve a power of 0.80 and a large effect size (1.2), a sample size of at least 105 is required, to detect a significant model. The transcriptions of the interviews and focus groups were analyzed via NVivo, using a thematic analysis [58]. A semantic approach was used, as opposed to a latent approach, to reduce the subjectivity of the researcher's judgment, and because the interest of this study is more based on people's stated experiences, rather than their assumptions. For the current article, qualitative data analysis was mainly used, to support the direction of the hypothesized associations, and to find out why certain hypothesized associations turned out to be insignificant.

2.4. Main Outcome Measures

We measured Sexual violence (SV) by asking respondents if they had ever experienced one of the following situations in the past two years ('No', 'Yes, once or twice', 'Yes, multiple times'). Those respondents answering 'Yes' to one of the 21 items were recoded as having experienced SV over the past two years. The World Health Organization's (2015) definition of SV was adopted, which includes different forms of sexual harassment without physical contact (hands-off SV), sexual abuse with physical contact but without penetration, and (attempted) rape (hands-on SV). Examples of items are 'Someone said I was sexually inept, abnormal, unattractive...', 'Someone stroked, rubbed, or touched the intimate parts of my body against my will (e.g., breasts, vagina, penis, anus)', and 'Someone inserted or tried to insert their penis, finger(s) or object(s) into my vagina or anus against my will'.

Quality of life was measured using Q4 from the Quality of Life Survey [26], which respondents answered, according to a 10-point Likert scale, with how satisfied they were with life right now, ranging from 'not at all satisfied' to 'very satisfied'.

Mental wellbeing was measured using the General Health Questionnaire 12 (GHQ-12, short version), in which 12 questions with four answer options were used to derive a total score on 12, in accordance with the Likert scoring method [59]. An example of a question is 'Have you lost confidence in yourself?' (with answer options: 'Not at all', 'Not more than usual', 'A little more than usual', and 'Much more than usual'). The higher the score, the lower wellbeing, or the higher the severity of psychological problems [60].

Participants were also asked a number of socio-demographic questions. Sexual orientation was measured by asking the respondents how they would describe their sexual orientation, with eight answer options: 'Heterosexual', 'Homosexual', 'Lesbian', 'Bi+', 'Asexual', 'Other', 'I don't know', and 'I don't want to say'. Based on the open answer responses to 'Other', the open answer 'Queer' was frequently mentioned, which led to the creation of an extra category. Respondents answering 'I don't want to say' were recoded as missing for this question. Sex assigned at birth (SAAB) was assessed with one question, asking respondents for their sex assigned at birth: 'Male', 'Female', 'Other', 'I don't want to say'.

The last two answer options were recoded as missing for this question. Gender identity was measured by asking all respondents how they would describe their gender identity at the current moment. A closed list of self-identification options was presented, from which they were asked to select only one option that fits them best: 'Man', 'Woman', 'Gender diverse (genderqueer, non-binary, agender, genderfluid, etc.)', 'Other', and 'I don't want to say'. If the SAAB was male and the gender identity woman, or if the SAAB was female and the gender identity was man, the respondent was recoded into the category Transgender. If the gender identity was gender-diverse, the respondent was recoded into Gender diverse (GD). Respondents registered the Region in which they currently lived, with the options 'Flemish Region', 'Brussels Capital Region', and 'Walloon Region (including the German-speaking community)'. The last option was recoded to missing, due to there being too small a sample size ($n = 5$). We measured the highest obtained educational level by asking about the highest level of education the participant had completed: 'Without diploma or primary education', 'Lower secondary education, general (3 first years completed)', 'Lower secondary education, technical/artistic/vocational (3 first years completed)', 'Higher secondary education, general (6 years completed)', 'Higher secondary education, technical/artistic (6 years completed)', 'Higher secondary education, vocational (6 years completed)', 'Higher education: graduate, candidacy, bachelor', 'University education: licentiate, postgraduate, master', 'Postgraduate', or 'Doctorate (PhD)'. The first six options were recoded to 'basic educational level', and the last four options to 'advanced educational level'. Work situation was assessed using a multiple response question about the respondent's current work situation. Respondents could reply to one or more of the following options: 'Student/in education', 'Unemployed/Looking for work', 'Long-term ill/incapacitated for work', 'Retired (also early retirement, pre-retirement)', 'Responsible for everyday shopping and taking care of the household', 'Employed (or temporary leave status)', 'I don't want to say'. This variable was recoded into a binary variable indicating whether or not someone is unemployed or long-term ill and not able to work, or employed/retired/taking care of the household. The last option was recoded to missing for this variable. Current relationship status was measured using one question, for which respondents had to choose one option that fitted them best: 'Single', 'I have a partner/partners but do not live with them', 'I am married or living together', 'I am divorced and not in a new relationship', 'I am a widow/widower and not in a new relationship', 'Other', or 'I don't want to say'. This variable was recoded into a binary variable with, on the one hand, all respondents indicating they are single, divorced, or a widower, and, on the other hand, all respondents currently in a relationship. Belonging to a minority group (ethnic–cultural, religious, disability status) was assessed using a question for which respondents had to indicate whether they belonged to the minority group ('Yes', 'No', 'I don't want to say'). For each minority group, respondents were recoded into a binary variable, indicating whether or not they belonged to the specific minority group ('Yes' or 'No'). The other respondents were recoded to missing. Age was recoded, after asking the respondent for their birth year. Economic vulnerability was measured using a question about how easily the respondents were able to make ends meet. The answer options ranged on a 6-point Likert scale from 'Very easy' to 'With great difficulty'. Hiding one's sexual orientation or changing one's physical appearance out of fear of getting attacked, discriminated against, or harassed, was assessed using a 4-point Likert scale, ranging from 'never' to 'always'.

3. Results

3.1. Study Sample and Characteristics

A total of 110 trans and GD youth between 15 and 25 years of age were included for data analyses. Four youths did not complete key survey items (e.g., sex assigned at birth or current gender identity), and were therefore not included in the final sample. The respondents' socio-demographic characteristics are summarized in Table 1. All the variables were dichotomized where possible (except for sexual orientation) and age, economic vulnerability, and both of the avoidance behaviors were used as continuous variables.

Table 1. Socio-demographic characteristics of the trans and gender-diverse sample (N = 110).

Variable Name	%	N
Gender identity		
Transgender	27.3	30
Gender diverse	72.7	80
Sexual orientation		
Heterosexual	3.6	4
Homosexual	7.3	8
Lesbian	15.5	17
Bi+	51.8	57
Asexual	8.2	9
Queer	11.8	13
I don't know yet	1.8	2
SAAB		
Female (AFAB)	82.2	88
Male (AMAB)	17.8	19
Region		
Flemish	97.3	107
Brussels Capital	2.7	3
Educational level		
Basic	42.7	47
Advanced	57.3	63
Work situation		
Student	75.5	83
Employed	16.4	18
Taking care of the household	1.8	2
Unemployed	8.2	9
Long-term ill	6.4	7
Relationship status		
Single	63.6	70
In a relationship	36.4	40
Minority status		
Ethnic–cultural	6.5	7
Religious	7.7	8
Disability	25	27
Economic vulnerability		
(Very) easily	40.4	44
Relatively easy/with a little effort	46.8	51
With (a lot of) difficulty	12.8	14

Table 1. Cont.

Variable Name	%	N
Hiding sexual orientation		
Never	19.8	19
Rarely	43.8	42
Often	34.4	33
Always	2.1	2
Changing physical appearance		
Never	13.1	14
Rarely	50.5	54
Often	31.8	34
Always	4.7	5
Age	M	SD
	20.0	3.0

Interview data from five trans and GD persons between 15 and 25 years of age were used. Most identified as non-binary ($n = 4$); one as a trans man. Four participants lived in the Flanders Region, and one in the Brussels Capital Region, and all participants were white. The youngest respondent was 19 years of age, and the oldest was 23 years of age.

3.2. Proportion of Sexual Violence

In total, 73.6% of the trans and GD adolescents and young adults reported having experienced sexual violence over the past two years ($n = 81$). Of these respondents, all reported hands-off sexual violence, with 60.5% of this group reporting at least one experience with hands-on sexual violence ($n = 49$). No significant difference in experiences with sexual violence was found between trans and GD respondents ($X^2(1) = 0.28, p = 0.60$). Economic vulnerability proved to be significantly associated with sexual violence ($p = 0.037$); trans and GD adolescents and young adults who had more difficulties making ends meet more frequently reported experiences with sexual violence.

3.3. Quality of Life (QoL) and Mental Wellbeing (GHQ-12)

The mean QoL for 15–25 year old trans and GD respondents was 5.4/10 ($SD = 1.93$). When comparing the respondents who experienced sexual violence in the past two years with those who did not, no significant difference in quality of life was found between victims and non-victims. However, when analyzing the association with the different socio-demographic background variables, a significant association was found between changing one's physical appearance out of fear of being attacked, discriminated against, or harassed, and quality of life. Trans and GD adolescents and young adults who indicated that they changed their physical appearance more often had a significant lower quality of life than those who did not. The other background variables were not significantly associated with QoL. See Table 2 for the ANCOVA results.

Table 2. ANCOVA analysis results for quality of life (QoL).

Variable	B	F	p	95% CI
Sexual violence (yes)	−0.58	2.03	0.157	[−1.39; 0.23]
Changing physical appearance	−0.64	7.08	0.009 **	[−1.12; −0.16]

Note: ** $p < 0.01$.

The Cronbach's alpha of the GHQ-12 scale within the sample was very good ($\alpha = 0.90$), with no item significantly improving the reliability statistic if deleted. The mean GHQ-12 score for 15–25 year old trans and GD respondents was 6.5/12 ($SD = 2.47$). When comparing the respondents who had experienced sexual violence in the past two years with those who had not, a marginally significant difference in mental wellbeing was found between victims and non-victims. When analyzing the association with the different socio-demographic background variables, a significant association was again found between changing one's physical appearance out of fear of being attacked, threatened, or harassed, and mental wellbeing. The more trans and GD adolescents and young adults changed their physical appearance out of fear, the higher the score on the GHQ-12, which indicates lower wellbeing or a higher severity of psychological problems. The other background variables were not significantly associated with the GHQ-12 score. See Table 3 for the ANCOVA results.

Table 3. ANCOVA analysis results for mental wellbeing (GHQ-12).

Variable	B	F	p	95% CI
Sexual violence (yes)	1.10	3.93	0.05	[−2.2; 0.002]
Changing physical appearance	0.69	4.29	0.041 *	[0.03; 1.34]

Note: * $p < 0.05$.

Due to the significant association between changing one's physical appearance and both the mental wellbeing outcome variables, the association between sexual violence and changing one's physical appearance was analyzed, to assess the possibility of an indirect effect of sexual violence on mental wellbeing (mediation). Results showed that trans and GD adolescents and young adults who had reported sexual violence in the past two years changed their physical appearance slightly more often, out of fear of being attacked, discriminated against, or harassed, than trans and GD non-victims. However, this association was not significant ($F(1,105) = 1.28$, $p = 0.261$).

3.4. Thematic Analysis of the Interviews and Focus Group

The thematic analysis of the transcripts of the interviews resulted in the identification of seven overarching themes: (1) experiences with sexual violence, (2) being trans or GD is experienced as a risk factor for sexual violence, (3) the negative emotional impact of violence, (4) fear and avoidance, (5) acceptance, (6) ignorance, and (7) mental health struggles not specifically related to violence. Some of these themes suggested a clearer picture of the association between sexual violence, changing one's physical appearance, and the two outcome variables (quality of life and mental wellbeing).

3.4.1. The Negative Emotional Impact of Violence

The direct impact of (sexual) violence on mental wellbeing is most obvious when taking a look at the emotions that respondents reported immediately after experiencing (sexual) violence. They mentioned feelings of gender dysphoria, loneliness, and inferiority. When asked about how they coped with their experiences, some mentioned that it left a permanent mark.

3.4.2. Fear and Avoidance

The long-term impact mentioned most often was fear of future violence and/or judgement. Many respondents reported trying to avoid violence and/or judgement. There were two main strategies: (1) some changed their expression (e.g., dressing differently to adhere to gender norms), and (2) some changed their behavior. These changes in behavior might have given respondents a sense of security, but they also inhibited them from practicing or receiving (self)care (e.g., stopping treatment for mental health problems, due to verbal violence from staff, or no longer going out for late-night mental-health walks, due to catcalling).

The interviews showed that sexual violence has an impact on how people present themselves to the public. However, this proved to be not only the case with victims of sexual violence. The anticipation and fear of sexual violence also caused trans and GD non-victims to behave and dress in a more gender-conforming way, which validates the non-significant association within the quantitative analyses.

4. Discussion

Incidents of sexual violence against trans and GD adolescents and young adults remain a reality, and multiple studies have found high proportions of sexual violence among trans and GD individuals. The proportion of sexual violence within the current study is 73.6%, which is a slightly higher proportion than the results found in the representative study of Keygnaert, De Schrijver, Cismaru Inescu, Schapansky, Nobels, Hahaut, Stappers, De Bauw, Lemonne, Renard, Weewauters, Nisen, Vander Beken and Vandeviver [32] (68%). Various studies highlight the association between sexual violence and age, with younger people reporting more sexual violence [25,32]. This could explain why the proportion is higher among trans and GD adolescents and young adults in the current study. However, The EU Agency for Fundamental Rights [25] showed that trans and GD individuals are at greater risk of experiencing sexual violence than other LGB+ groups. The study of Keygnaert, De Schrijver, Cismaru Inescu, Schapansky, Nobels, Hahaut, Stappers, De Bauw, Lemonne, Renard, Weewauters, Nisen, Vander Beken and Vandeviver [32] addressed sexual violence among LGBTI+ people, and the proportion of trans and GD respondents in the sample was very low (1.7%), which might also explain the lower proportion of sexual violence within this study. Future research assessing experiences with sexual violence in this group, using the same conceptualization of sexual violence, and examining the same age group, will provide more insight into the representativeness of the results.

The mental wellbeing of trans and GD adolescents and young adults is also lower, compared to existing European and Belgian statistics. The mean score for quality of life (QoL) was 5.3/10, which is in line with the results of the EU Agency for Fundamental Rights [29], which showed that trans and GD individuals aged 15–25 had an average QoL of 5.2/10. The results are much lower than the average QoL score in the general Belgian population aged 18–24, which is 7.6/10 [26]. The trans and GD adolescents and young adults within the current study appear to have a much lower mental wellbeing, or a higher severity of psychological problems, in comparison with the general Belgian population. The average GHQ-12 score within the current study was 6.6/12, which is much higher than the average of 1.3/12 in the general Belgian population [27], and even much higher than the average score found by Motmans, T'Sjoen and Meier [2], measured among trans respondents (3.9/12).

When the association between sexual violence and both of the wellbeing scores was assessed, only a marginally significant association between sexual violence and the GHQ-12 score could be found ($p = 0.50$). None of the background variables seemed to be significantly associated with either of the mental wellbeing outcome variables, except for changing one's appearance out of fear of being attacked, discriminated against, or harassed. Trans and GD adolescents and young adults who indicated that they changed their appearance more often had a significantly lower QoL ($p = 0.009$), and a significantly higher GHQ-12 score ($p = 0.041$). The high proportion of sexual violence, as well as the lower average QoL and higher average GHQ-12 scores, among trans and GD adolescents and young adults, compared to general population statistics, highlights the need for policy makers to create more inclusive environments.

The current study provides some validation of the theory of violence, and gender nonconformity as a motive for violence [2,7,25,40,41,45,46]. In accordance with the Minority Stress Theory, trans and GD individuals develop a fear of experiencing violence, based on awareness of existing stigma and actual experiences with violence [17–21]. In anticipating future violence, trans and GD adolescents and young adults indicated that they would modify their appearance to conform to the prevailing binary gender norms, regardless of whether they had been victims of sexual violence in the past. Based on the interviews, it became clear that trans and GD individuals who adapted their appearance more often did not necessarily experience more violence. They indicated that they adapted their appearance out of fear of future victimization. This also validates the non-significant association between sexual violence and gender nonconformity within the quantitative data analyses ($p = 0.261$).

One of the limitations of the current study is that the sampling strategy may have produced skewed data. A convenience sampling strategy was used to collect data. This means that it cannot be guaranteed that the results obtained are representative of the entire Flemish trans and GD community between the age of 15–25. The survey was mainly distributed using posters, flyers, and social media. The posters and flyers were mainly distributed during LGBTI+ events, and in urban areas. Individuals living in rural areas may not have been reached. Furthermore, the quantitative data were gathered online, so respondents were expected to have digital literacy. Nevertheless, the results provide an indicator of what is going on within the Flemish young trans and GD community.

In the past two decades, a number of studies have assessed experiences with violence among trans and GD people. However, a number of references within this article refer to studies from the 1980s and 1990s. Replication of these studies should be performed, to confirm that the theories behind the motives of violence still apply.

5. Conclusions

Sexual violence is a common reality among trans and GD adolescents and young adults. The literature has already indicated that people who challenge gender norms are much more visible, and therefore also much more vulnerable. Observing gender-non-conforming behavior can lead to violent behavior. Trans and gender-diverse people do not always fit the binary male/female framework, meaning that a discrepancy between their appearance and their sex assigned at birth can provoke violence. Therefore, awareness campaigns should pay more attention to themes such as gender identity and gender expression. These themes should be included in various training courses, and broader campaigns on violence.

The present study suggests that it is not sexual violence per se that leads to poorer wellbeing. What appears to be more important is the tendency to adapt one's appearance to be more gender conforming that leads to a lower QoL and GhQ-12 score. Gender nonconformity appears to be an important factor in mental wellbeing. Trans and GD adolescents and young adults who indicated that they adjusted their appearance more often to conform to the binary gender roles in society, out of fear of getting attacked, discriminated against, or harassed, had significantly lower QoL, and a significantly higher GHQ-21 score. We emphasize that these associations are not limited to sexual violence victims, but appear to be similar for both victims and non-victims. The anticipation of future sexual violence leads people to change their appearance, to be more gender conforming. Future studies should try to disentangle the possible reasons behind the association of gender nonconformity and wellbeing.

Author Contributions: Conceptualization, A.B. and J.M.; methodology, A.B.; software, A.B. and J.V.W.; validation, A.B. and J.V.W.; formal analysis, A.B. and J.V.W.; investigation, A.B. and J.V.W.; resources, A.B.; data curation, A.B.; writing—original draft preparation, A.B.; writing—review and editing, A.B.; visualization, A.B.; supervision, J.M.; project administration, J.M.; funding acquisition, A.B. and J.M. All authors have read and agreed to the published version of the manuscript.

Funding: This research was funded by the Flemish Government, grant number ABB/GKII/GK/2020/002.

Institutional Review Board Statement: The study was conducted in accordance with the Declaration of Helsinki, and approved by the Ethics Committee of Ghent University Hospital (protocol code BC-10233, approved on 10 September 2021).

Informed Consent Statement: Informed consent was obtained from all subjects involved in the study.

Data Availability Statement: The data presented in this study are available on request from the corresponding author. The data are not publicly available due to the fact that the dataset contains personal data.

Conflicts of Interest: The authors declare no conflict of interest.

References

1. D'haese, L.; Dewaele, A.; Van Houtte, M. Geweld Tegenover Holebi's II: Een Online Survey over Ervaringen Met Holebigeweld in Vlaanderen en de Nasleep Ervan. S. Gelijkekansenbeleid. 2014. Available online: http://www.steunpuntgelijkekansen.be/wp-content/uploads/Geweld-tegenover-Holebis-II-tussentijdsrapport-2014-Lies-dHaese-130514-bvl.pdf (accessed on 15 May 2023).
2. Motmans, J.; T'Sjoen, G.; Meier, P. Geweldervaringen van Transgender Personen in België. G. Kansenbeleid. 2015. Available online: https://www.researchgate.net/publication/279033654_Geweldervaringen_van_transgender_personen_in_Belgie (accessed on 15 May 2023).
3. Burke, S.E.; Dovidio, J.F.; Przedworski, J.M.; Hardeman, R.R.; Perry, S.P.; Phelan, S.M.; Nelson, D.B.; Burgess, D.J.; Yeazel, M.W.; van Ryn, M. Do contact and empathy mitigate bias against gay and lesbian people among heterosexual first-year medical students? A report from the medical student CHANGE study. *Acad. Med.* **2015**, *90*, 645–651. [CrossRef] [PubMed]
4. European Commission. Special Eurobarometer 493: Discrimination in the European Union. 2019. Available online: https://europa.eu/eurobarometer/surveys/detail/2251 (accessed on 15 May 2023).
5. Herek, G.M.; Capitanio, J.P. "Some of My Best Friends": Intergroup Contact, ConcealableStigma, and Heterosexuals' Attitudes Toward Gay Men and Lesbians. *Personal. Soc. Psychol. Bull.* **1996**, *22*, 412–424. [CrossRef]
6. Hooghe, M.; Quintelier, E.; Claes, E.; Dejaeghere, Y.; Harrell, A. *De Houding van Jongeren ten Aanzien van Holebi-Rechten: Een Kwantitatieve en Kwalitatieve Analyse*; Centrum voor Politicologie: Leuven, Belgium, 2007.
7. Buijs, L.; Hekma, G.; Duyvendak, J. Als ze Maar van me Afblijven: Een Onderzoek naar Antihomoseksueel Geweld in Amsterdam. 2009. Available online: https://library.oapen.org/viewer/web/viewer.html?file=/bitstream/handle/20.500.12657/35266/340064.pdf?sequence=1&isAllowed=y (accessed on 13 July 2022).
8. D'Augelli, A.R. Developmental implications of victimization of lesbian, gay, and bisexual youths. In *Stigma and Sexual Orientation: Understanding Prejudice against Lesbians, Gay Men, and Bisexuals*; Herek, G.M., Ed.; Sage Publications: New York, NY, USA, 1998; pp. 187–201.
9. D'Augelli, A.R.; Grossman, A.H. Disclosure of sexual orientation, victimization, and mental health among lesbian, gay, and bisexual older adults. *J. Interpers. Violence* **2001**, *16*, 1008–1027. [CrossRef]
10. Katz-Wise, S.L.; Hyde, J.S. Victimization experiences of lesbian, gay, and bisexual individuals: A meta-analysis. *J. Sex Res.* **2012**, *49*, 142–167. [CrossRef] [PubMed]
11. Pilkington, N.W.; D'Augelli, A.R. Victimization of lesbian, gay, and bisexual youth in community settings. *J. Community Psychol.* **1995**, *23*, 33–56. [CrossRef]
12. Coleman, E.; Radix, A.E.; Bouman, W.P.; Brown, G.R.; de Vries, A.L.C.; Deutsch, M.B.; Ettner, R.; Fraser, L.; Goodman, M.; Green, J.; et al. Standards of Care for the Health of Transgender and Gender Diverse People, Version 8. *Int. J. Transgender Health* **2022**, *23*, S1–S259. [CrossRef]
13. Meyer, I.H. Minority Stress and Mental Health in Gay Men. *J. Health Soc. Behav.* **1995**, *36*, 38. [CrossRef]
14. Meyer, I.H. Prejudice, social stress, and mental health in lesbian, gay, and bisexual populations: Conceptual issues and research evidence. *Psychol. Bull.* **2003**, *129*, 674–697. [CrossRef]
15. Dentato, M.P. The Minority Stress Perspective. Minority Stress Is the Relationship between Minority and Dominant Values and Resultant Conflict with the Social Environment Experienced by Minority Group Members. Psychology and AIDS Exchange Newsletter. 2012. Available online: https://www.apa.org/pi/aids/resources/exchange/2012/04/minority-stress (accessed on 15 May 2023).
16. Marshal, M.P.; Friedman, M.S.; Stall, R.; King, K.M.; Miles, J.; Gold, M.A.; Bukstein, O.G.; Morse, J.Q. Sexual orientation and adolescent substance use: A meta-analysis and methodological review. *Addiction* **2008**, *103*, 546–556. [CrossRef]
17. Johnson, K.; Auerswald, C.; LeBlanc, A.J.; Bockting, W.O. Invalidation Experiences and Protective Factors Among Non-Binary Adolescents. *J. Adolesc. Health* **2019**, *64*, S4. [CrossRef]
18. Kelleher, C. Minority stress and health: Implications for lesbian, gay, bisexual, transgender, and questioning (LGBTQ) young people. *Couns. Psychol. Q.* **2009**, *22*, 373–379. [CrossRef]
19. Mackenzie, S. Experiences of Gender and Sexual Minority Stress Among LGBTQ Families: The Role of Community Resilience and Minority Coping. In *Sexual and Gender Minority Health*; Emerald Publishing Limited: Bingley, UK, 2021; pp. 181–206. [CrossRef]
20. Rood, B.A.; Reisner, S.L.; Surace, F.I.; Puckett, J.A.; Maroney, M.R.; Pantalone, D.W. Expecting Rejection: Understanding the Minority Stress Experiences of Transgender and Gender-Nonconforming Individuals. *Transgender Health* **2016**, *1*, 151–164. [CrossRef]
21. Testa, R.J.; Habarth, J.; Peta, J.; Balsam, K.; Bockting, W. Development of the Gender Minority Stress and Resilience Measure. *Psychol. Sex. Orientat. Gend. Divers.* **2015**, *2*, 65–78. [CrossRef]
22. Testa, R.J.; Michaels, M.S.; Bliss, W.; Rogers, M.L.; Balsam, K.F.; Joiner, T. Suicidal ideation in transgender people: Gender minority stress and interpersonal theory factors. *J. Abnorm. Psychol.* **2017**, *126*, 125–136. [CrossRef]

23. Aparicio-García, M.; Díaz-Ramiro, E.; Rubio-Valdehita, S.; López-Núñez, M.; García-Nieto, I. Health and Well-Being of Cisgender, Transgender and Non-Binary Young People. *Int. J. Environ. Res. Public Health* **2018**, *15*, 2133. [CrossRef]
24. Bränström, R.; Stormbom, I.; Bergendal, M.; Pachankis, J.E. Transgender-based disparities in suicidality: A population-based study of key predictions from four theoretical models. *Suicide Life-Threat. Behav.* **2022**, *52*, 401–412. [CrossRef]
25. EU Agency for Fundamental Rights. *A Long Way to Go for LGBTI Equality*; Publications Office of the European Union: Luxembourg, 2020; Available online: https://fra.europa.eu/sites/default/files/fra_uploads/fra-2020-lgbti-equality-1_en.pdf (accessed on 15 April 2023).
26. Eurofound. *European Quality of Life Survey 2016: Quality of Life, Quality of Public Services, and Quality of Society*; Publications Office of the European Union: Luxembourg, 2017.
27. Gisle, L. Gezondheidsenquête, België. 2018. Available online: https://www.sciensano.be/sites/default/files/1-mental_health_report_2018_nl2.pdf (accessed on 15 May 2023).
28. Howell, J.; Maguire, R. Seeking help when transgender: Exploring the difference in mental and physical health seeking behaviors between transgender and cisgender individuals in Ireland. *Int. J. Transgenderism* **2019**, *20*, 421–433. [CrossRef] [PubMed]
29. EU Agency for Fundamental Rights. LGBTI Survey Data Explorer. 2020. Available online: https://fra.europa.eu/en/data-and-maps/2020/lgbti-survey-data-explorer (accessed on 23 March 2023).
30. Basile, K.C.; Smith, S.G.; Breiding, M.; Black, M.C.; Mahendra, R.R. Sexual Violence Surveillance: Uniform Definitions and Recommended Data Elements. Version 2.0. 2014. Available online: https://stacks.cdc.gov/view/cdc/26326#:~:text=Sexual%20Violence%20Surveillance%3A%20Uniform%20Definitions%20and%20Recommended%20Data,document%20was%20developed%20through%20an%20extensive%20consultation%20process (accessed on 23 March 2023).
31. Krahé, B.; Tomaszewska, P.; Kuyper, L.; Vanwesenbeeck, I. Prevalence of sexual aggression among young people in Europe: A review of the evidence from 27 EU countries. *Agression Violent Behav.* **2014**, *19*, 545–558. [CrossRef]
32. Keygnaert, I.; De Schrijver, L.; Cismaru Inescu, A.; Schapansky, E.; Nobels, A.; Hahaut, B.; Stappers, C.; De Bauw, Z.; Lemonne, A.; Renard, B.; et al. UN-MENAMAIS: Understanding the Mechanisms, Nature, Magnitude and Impact of Sexual Violence in Belgium. 2021. Available online: http://www.belspo.be/belspo/brain-be/projects/FinalReports/UN-MENAMAIS_FinalRep_v2.pdf (accessed on 25 August 2022).
33. World Health Organization. Strengthening the Medico-Legal Response to Sexual Violence. 2015. Available online: https://reliefweb.int/report/world/strengthening-medico-legal-response-sexual-violence#:~:text=A%20strong%20medico-legal%20response%20is%20necessary%20to%20help,investigation%2C%20and%20ethical%20standards%20that%20must%20be%20upheld (accessed on 23 March 2023).
34. D'Augelli, A.R.; Pilkington, N.W.; Hershberger, S.L. Incidence and mental health impact of sexual orientation victimization of lesbian, gay, and bisexual youths in high school. *Sch. Psychol. Q.* **2002**, *17*, 148–167. [CrossRef]
35. Felten, H.; Schuyf, J. Zoenen Is Gevaarlijk. Onderzoek Naar Geweld Tegen lesBische Vrouwen. 2011. Available online: https://www.movisie.nl/sites/movisie.nl/files/publication-attachment/Rapport%20onderzoek%20naar%20geweld%20tegen%20lesBische%20vrouwen%20%5BMOV-181998-0.3%5D.pdf (accessed on 15 May 2023).
36. Garnets, L.; Herek, G.M.; Levy, B. Violence and Victimization of Lesbians and Gay Men. *J. Interpers. Violence* **1990**, *5*, 366–383. [CrossRef]
37. Willis, D.G. Meanings in adult male victims' experiences of hate crime and its aftermath. *Issues Ment. Health Nurs.* **2008**, *29*, 567–584. [CrossRef] [PubMed]
38. Walters, M.A.; Paterson, J.; Brown, R.; McDonnell, L. Hate Crimes Against Trans People: Assessing Emotions, Behaviors, and Attitudes Toward Criminal Justice Agencies. *J. Interpers. Violence* **2017**, *35*, 4583–4613. [CrossRef] [PubMed]
39. HRC Foundation. Glossary of Terms. 2022. Available online: https://www.hrc.org/resources/glossary-of-terms (accessed on 30 May 2023).
40. Blondeel, K.; De Vasconcelos, S.; García-Moreno, C.; Stephenson, R.; Temmerman, M.; Toskin, I. Violence motivated by perception of sexual orientation and gender identity: A systematic review. *Bull. World Health Organ.* **2017**, *96*, 29–41. [CrossRef]
41. Ortiz-Hernández, L.; Torres, M.I.G. Efectos de la violencia y la discriminación en la salud mental de bisexuales, lesbianas y homosexuales de la Ciudad de México. *Cad. de Saúde Pública* **2005**, *21*, 913–925. [CrossRef] [PubMed]
42. Gordon, A.R.; Meyer, I.H. Gender Nonconformity as a Target of Prejudice, Discrimination, and Violence Against LGB Individuals. *J. LGBT Health Res.* **2007**, *3*, 55–71. [CrossRef]
43. Herek, G.M. The social context of hate crimes: Notes on cultural heterosexism. In *Hate Crimes: Confronting Violence against Lesbians and Gay Men*; Herek, G.M., Berrill, K.T., Eds.; Sage Publications: New York, NY, USA, 1992; pp. 89–104.
44. Herek, G.M. Gender Gaps in Public Opinion about Lesbians and Gay Men. *Public Opin. Q.* **2002**, *66*, 40–66. [CrossRef]
45. Turner, L.; Whittle, S.; Combs, R. Transphobic Hate Crime in the European Union. 2009. Available online: https://transgenderinfo.be/wp-content/uploads/transphobic_hate_crime_in_eu.pdf (accessed on 13 July 2022).
46. D'Augelli, A.R.; Grossman, A.H.; Starks, M.T. Childhood gender atypicality, victimization, and PTSD among lesbian, gay, and bisexual youth. *J. Interpers. Violence* **2006**, *2*, 1462–1482. [CrossRef]
47. Chamberland, L. *The Impact of Homophobia and Homophobic Violence on the Perseverance and Scholar Success*; Université du Québec à Montréal: Montreal, QC, Canada, 2011.
48. Testa, R.J.; Sciacca, L.M.; Wang, F.; Hendricks, M.L.; Goldblum, P.; Bradford, J.; Bongar, B. Effects of violence on transgender people. *Prof. Psychol. Res. Pract.* **2012**, *43*, 452–459. [CrossRef]

49. D'haese, L.; Dewaele, A.; Van Houtte, M. The Relationship Between Childhood Gender Nonconformity and Experiencing Diverse Types of Homophobic Violence. *J. Interpers. Violence* **2015**, *31*, 1634–1660. [CrossRef]
50. Agler, R.; De Boeck, P. On the Interpretation and Use of Mediation: Multiple Perspectives on Mediation Analysis. *Front. Psychol.* **2017**, *8*, 1984. [CrossRef] [PubMed]
51. Hayes, A.F. *Introduction to Mediation, Moderation, and Conditional Process Analysis: A Regression-Based Approach*; The Guilford Press: New York, NY, USA, 2013.
52. O'Rourke, H.P.; MacKinnon, D.P. Reasons for Testing Mediation in the Absence of an Intervention Effect: A Research Imperative in Prevention and Intervention Research. *Stud. Alcohol Drugs* **2018**, *79*, 171–181. [CrossRef] [PubMed]
53. IBM Corp. *IBM SPSS Statistics for Windows, Version 28.0*; IBM SPSS: Armonk, NY, USA, 2021.
54. Chow, S.; Shao, J.; Wang, H.; Lokhnygina, Y. *Sample Size Calculations in Clinical Research*; Chapman and Hall/CRC: Boca Raton, FL, USA, 2017. [CrossRef]
55. Cohen, J. *Statistical Power Analysis for the Behavioral Sciences*; Lawrence Erlbaum Associates: Mahwah, NJ, USA, 1988. [CrossRef]
56. Hsieh, F.Y.; Bloch, D.A.; Larsen, M.D. A simple method of sample size calculation for linear and logistic regression. *Stat. Med.* **1998**, *17*, 1623–1634. [CrossRef]
57. Hulley, S.B.; Cummings, S.R.; Browner, W.S.; Hearst, N.; Grady, D.; Newman, T.B. *Designing Clinical Research: An Epidemiologic Approach*; Lippincott Williams & Wilkins: Philadelphia, PA, USA, 2001.
58. QSR International Pty Ltd. *NVivo Qualitative Data Analysis Software*. Version 12. 2018. Available online: https://www.qsrinternational.com/nvivo-qualitative-data-analysis-software/home (accessed on 10 July 2023).
59. Goldberg, D.P.; McDowell, I.; Newell, C. General health questionnaire (GHQ), 12 item version, 20 item version, 30 item version, 60 item version [GHQ12, GHQ20, GHQ30, GHQ60]. In *Measuring Health: A Guide Rotating Scales and Questionnaire*; Oxford University Press: Oxford, UK, 1972; pp. 225–236.
60. Goldberg, D.; Willimas, P. A User's Guide to the General Health Questionnaire. 1988. Available online: https://cir.nii.ac.jp/crid/1130000795003754752 (accessed on 2 August 2022).

Disclaimer/Publisher's Note: The statements, opinions and data contained in all publications are solely those of the individual author(s) and contributor(s) and not of MDPI and/or the editor(s). MDPI and/or the editor(s) disclaim responsibility for any injury to people or property resulting from any ideas, methods, instructions or products referred to in the content.

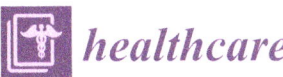

Review

Risk Factors Linked to Violence in Female Same-Sex Couples in Hispanic America: A Scoping Review

Leonor Garay-Villarroel [1], Angela Castrechini-Trotta [1,2,*] and Immaculada Armadans-Tremolosa [1,2]

[1] Department of Social Psychology and Quantitative Psychology, University of Barcelona, 08035 Barcelona, Spain; lgarayvi7@alumnes.ub.edu (L.G.-V.); iarmadans@ub.edu (I.A.-T.)
[2] PsicoSAO—Research Group in Social, Environmental and Organizational Psychology, University of Barcelona, 08035 Barcelona, Spain
* Correspondence: acastrechini@ub.edu

Abstract: Intimate partner violence (IPV) among women is an understudied topic in Hispanic Americans; therefore, we aim to describe this phenomenon and its associated risk factors in comparison with other sexual orientations and practices. A scoping review was carried out using the following databases: Scopus, Web of Science, Redalyc, Scielo.org, and Dialnet. The following keywords were used: same-sex, intragender, couple, domestic, and partner violence. The inclusion criteria applied were studies published between 2000 and 2022 with a minimum participation of 15% of Hispanic Americans, resulting in 23 articles. The findings showed a lower presence of studies on violence in women compared to men. Minority stress, power dynamics, social support, and childhood experiences of violence, which are related and complementary to each other, were identified as risk factors. We concluded that there is little research on IPV among women. In addition, studies require a renewed focus to comprehend this type of violence, which cannot be equated with those of heterosexual couples. This approach continues to perpetuate the invisibility of this problem, and, therefore, a more inclusive and specific perspective is needed.

Keywords: female same-sex couples; violence; risks factors; scoping review

1. Introduction

Intimate partner violence (IPV) is an important public health issue [1–3]. However, IPV among female same-sex couples (FSSC) is a complex and understudied problem in the context of Hispanic America (Spanish-speaking countries in the Americas). Although there has been progress and research on this topic, it is essential to deepen an understanding of properly addressing risk factors and establishing effective measures for prevention and care.

IPV among FSSC is currently a problem of considerable magnitude [4,5] due to its invisibility. It has been shown that the incidence of violence in female couples is comparable and even higher than that occurring in heterosexual relationships [6–8].

It is important to stress that the term "FSSC" is used in this research in order to include diverse orientations and practices within this category (lesbian couples, bisexual women, pansexual women, etc.).

IPV is defined as a set of behaviors that encompasses physical violence, stalking, and psychological aggression, including coercive tactics. These behaviors are carried out by a current or former intimate partner, such as spouses, girlfriends, or sexual partners [2].

Currently, IPV among FSSCs is socially invisible. One reason could be gender norms, as there is a social perception that women are less likely to use violence as a means of personal communication [5].

There is little research on IPV in women involved in same-sex relationships [9,10] and the risk factors that interact with this phenomenon, especially in a Hispanic American context.

A study by Swan and colleagues [11] found that a little over half of the participants in their sample had experienced some form of IPV victimization at some point in their lives, while slightly more than half had taken part in at least one form of perpetration. Among these cases, psychological aggression emerged as the most common type of victimization and perpetration.

To understand IPV in this population group, it is important to address risk factors, defined as those individual, environmental, sociocultural, economic, and/or behavioral factors that could generate adverse consequences [12,13].

In IPV, the impact of risk factors is not isolated, and they can converge from various contexts; therefore, the ecological model of Bronfenbrenner [14] is useful for its study. This model proposes that the conduct and behavior of people are a set of structures organized at different levels that are linked to each other. Therefore, violence could be linked from very early stages to adulthood [15]. In addition, the variables that contribute to violence are found at different interrelated levels. These levels include the macrosocial level (within a given culture or sub-culture), the exosystem (one or more environments where the person is not included), the mesosystem (interrelationship of two or more environments, or networks), as well as the microsystem (close environment) [14].

It is important to consider new ways of understanding violence, especially in relationships between women. This involves addressing the macrostructural context, such as the stress experienced by minorities [16], which refers to the excess stress that individuals belonging to stigmatized social categories face due to their social position, sometimes in minority circumstances [16]. When comparing the levels of minority stressors in some cases, lesbians exhibit a greater anticipation of rejection compared to gay individuals [17]. Additionally, individuals who frequently report experiencing discrimination in public spaces also simultaneously indicate a certain degree of internalized homophobia [18].

Within this context, there is a specific form of violence known as "identity abuse" (IA), which involves an abusive tactic used within an intimate partnership, leveraging the oppression of systems such as ableism, heterosexism, sexism, and racism to harm the partner [19,20]. However, very few studies have addressed this aspect in violent female-to-female relationships.

All in all, the importance of detecting the risk factors associated with IPV among women involved in same-sex relationships in Hispanic America lies in generating better prevention and care strategies for affected communities. Therefore, this scoping review focuses on research published from 2000 to 2022 with the purpose of describing two relevant aspects. The first aspect aims to contextualize the prevalence of studies involving couples of women who have experienced violence in comparison to other intragender relationships. The second aspect involves identifying the risk factors associated with violence in FSSC.

2. Materials and Methods

2.1. Design

The study involved a scoping review: a systematic knowledge synthesis method used to comprehensively represent evidence on a topic. This approach aims to identify essential concepts, including theories, sources, and knowledge gaps [21]. In the specific context of our research, it effectively synthesized evidence concerning violence within women's relationships. This was of particular significance due to the diverse range of findings within the chosen studies. Given the study's objective and the preliminary investigation conducted on this topic, the scoping review was deemed a suitable approach. This is because it serves as an optimal mechanism to ascertain the extent or breadth of the literature pertaining to a specific subject, offering a comprehensive overview of the volume of the literature and studies accessible, along with a broad or detailed depiction of its focal points [21–23]. The steps followed by this study consisted of designing the research question, elaborating the search strategies based on keywords, selecting the databases, establishing the inclusion and exclusion criteria, selecting articles for review, creating categories to guide the analysis, and, finally, conducting the analysis of the selected articles and producing the results.

As a search strategy we used the PRISMA Extension for Scoping Reviews (PRISMA-ScR) [21] with the purpose of describing the prevalence of studies on intimate partner violence among women in Hispanic America in relation to other sexual orientations/practices, and the main associated risk factors.

2.2. Search Method

For this study, we searched for articles in the Scopus, Web of Science, Redalyc, Scielo.org, and Dialnet databases. The criterion for choosing the databases was based on the selection of databases used and recognized at an academic level, both worldwide and in Latin America. The keywords used in English had the following combinations: same sex AND couple violence; same-sex AND partner violence; intragender AND partner violence; intragender AND couple violence; intragender AND domestic violence; intra-gender AND partner violence; intra-gender AND couple violence; intra-gender AND domestic violence; same-sex AND domestic violence; same-sex AND couple violence; same-sex AND partner violence; same-sex AND couple violence.

In Spanish, the keywords were: Violencia en parejas del mismo sexo; violencia doméstica en parejas del mismo sexo; violencia en parejas intragénero; violencia en parejas LGTBI; violencia en parejas del mismo género.

2.3. Inclusion and Exclusion Criterion

- The inclusion criteria:
    1. Studies whose main purpose was to analyze violence in couples.
    2. Studies published between 2000 and 2022.
    3. Studies that included the LGTBIQ+ population as the main sample.
    4. Studies in English and Spanish *.
    5. Journal articles that had undergone peer review (to ensure the quality of the publication).
    6. Studies with a minimum of 15% of participants/a Spanish–American sample *.
    7. Studies that included only participants over 18.

* Due to these criteria, the study is classified as Hispanic American rather than Latin American, as Portuguese literature was not taken into consideration

- Exclusion criteria (failure to comply with one of these criteria means that the publication is excluded):
    1. Theoretical articles, systematic reviews, meta-analyses, and trials.
    2. Articles in which the main purpose is not to measure IPV.
    3. Articles that do not have a Hispanic American population.
    4. Articles that include participants under 18.
    5. Non-blind peer-reviewed publications.
    6. Articles written in languages other than Spanish or English.

The search of the database yielded 851 articles, and after the elimination of duplicate studies, a total of 276 articles were obtained. The inclusion and exclusion criteria were applied to these articles based on the review of the title and abstract, leaving 27 records for the complete review, of which four were discarded due to failure to meet the criteria, including underage participants, participants with results in the process, and studies that did not have a minimum of 15% of Hispanic American participants. Finally, the publications selected for the review and analysis equaled 23 (see Figure 1).

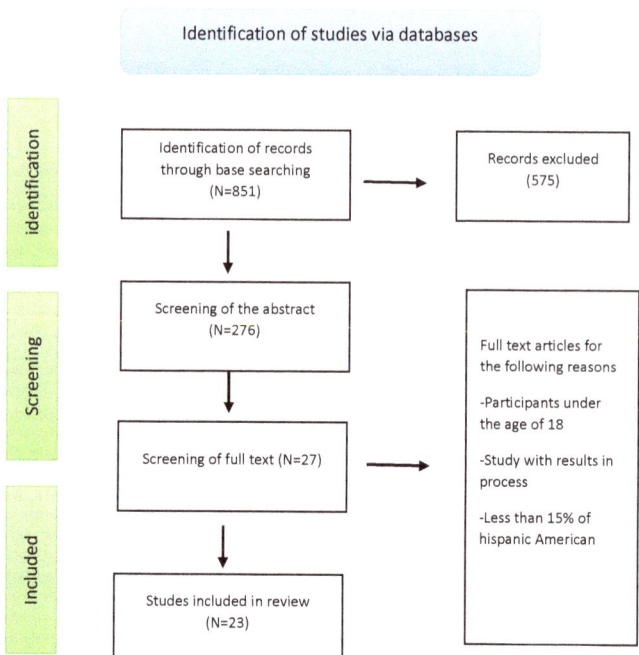

Figure 1. PRISMA flow diagram.

Additionally, Figure 2 displays the number of articles located in each database, clarifying that some articles appeared in more than one database.

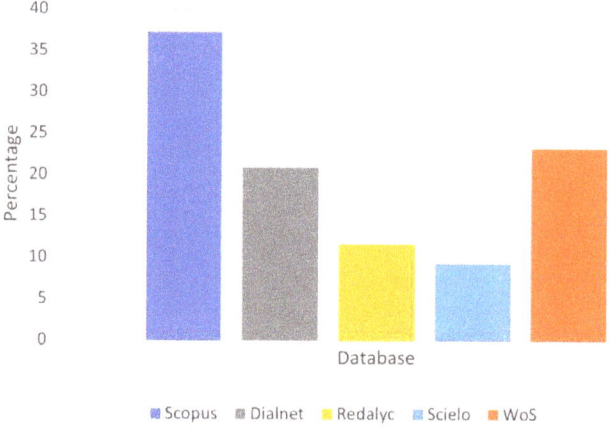

Figure 2. Distribution of articles based on scientific databases. Note: WoS: Web of Science.

The selected studies were analyzed in detail, considering both their relevance to the review and their methodological reliability.

2.4. Data Extraction

The first part corresponded to the registration of the articles found in the databases. To organize and categorize the information, manual tables were prepared in Excel containing the following aspects: the name of the publication, year, database from which it was extracted, journal, language, country, keywords, population, methodology, and summary.

For the second part, which corresponded to the analysis of the selected articles, the Atlas-ti 9 program was used to deepen the contents and draw up maps of the relationships.

2.5. Data Analysis and Synthesis of Results

Once the data were organized in the Excel document, descriptive statistics were used to present some of the features of the included studies. A thematic analysis [24] was then performed to summarize the findings according to the research purpose. Both the categories and their results were compared among the reviewers, and disagreements were worked out until a consensus was reached.

3. Results

To describe the results, first, an overview was conducted to contextualize the current state of intragender IPV research with Hispanic American participants, paying particular attention to the frequency of studies focused on female couples. Second, the main risk factors associated with IPV among women were identified and analyzed.

3.1. Comparing Studies Focusing on FSSC with Other Intragender Relationships

Regarding violence in same-sex couples, a larger number of quantitative studies (n = 17) [25–41] compared to qualitative (n = 5) [42–46] were found, with only one mixed study [47] (see Table 1).

Table 1. Overview of the studies.

Article	Method	Country of First Author	Origin of Participants	Sexual Orientation/Sexual Practice
Barrientos et al. [25]	Quantitative	Chile	Spain 399 (63.3%) Mexico 130 (20.6%) Venezuela 57 (9%) Chile 44 (7%)	Lesbians 285 (45.2%) Gays 345 (54.7%)
Bosco et al. [26]	Quantitative	USA	White E/C 225 (66.4%) Black/Afro 27 (8.0%) Hispanos 51 (15.0%) Other 36 (10.6%)	Gays 304 (87.7%) Bisexual men 35 (10.3%)
L. Rodríguez & Lara. [27]	Quantitative	Mexico	Mexico 277 (100%)	Homosexual 128 (64.6%) Heterosexual 49 (24.7%) Bisexuals 20 (10.1%) Other 1 (0.5%)
Redondo-Pacheco et al. [28]	Quantitative	Colombia	Colombia 132 (100%)	Gays 93 (70.5%) Lesbians 39 (29.5%)
Longares et al. [29]	Quantitative	Spain	Spain (44.6%) Mexico (20%) Venezuela (8.5%) Chile (8.5%)	Gays 147 (48.2%) Lesbians 112 (36.7%) Pansexual or bisexual 46 (15.1%)
Davis et al. [30]	Quantitative	USA	White E/C 85 (45%) Asian 6 (3.2%) Hispano 39 (20.6%) Black/Afro 49 (25.9%) Other 9 (4.8%)	MSM 189 (100%)

Table 1. Cont.

Article	Method	Country of First Author	Origin of Participants	Sexual Orientation/Sexual Practice
Stephenson et al. [31]	Quantitative	USA	White E/C 191 (47.67%) Black/Afro 60 (14.86%) Hispanic 151 (37.47%)	Bisexual 77 (19.07%) Homosexual 325 (80.93%)
Reyes et al. [32]	Quantitative	Puerto Rico	Puerto Rico 201 (100%)	Gays 124 (61.7%) Lesbians 66 (32.8%) Bisexual women 6 (3%) Bisexual men 5 (2.5%)
Loveland & Raghavan. [33]	Quantitative	USA	White E/C (8.1%) Black/Afro (49.3%) Hispanos (21.3%) Other (21.3%)	Gay 24 (17%) Bisexual men 32 (24.4%) Not identified 22 (16.3%) Heterosexual men 24 (17.8%) MSM 34 (24.5%)
Houston & McKirnan. [34]	Quantitative	USA	White E/C 182 (22.4%) Black/Afro 419 (51.3%) Hispanos 133 (16.3%) Asian/Pacific islanders or other ethnicities 82 (10%)	Gays 609 (74.5%) Bisexual men 104 (12.7%) MSM 104 (12.8%)
Gómez et al. [35]	Quantitative	Chile	Chile 467 (100%)	Lesbians 199 (42.6%) Gays 268 (57.4%)
S. Rodríguez & Toro-Alfonso. [36]	Quantitative	Puerto Rico	Puerto Rico 302 (100%)	Gays 245 (81%) Bisexual men 57 (19%)
McLaughlin & Rozee. [37]	Quantitative	USA	White E/C 151 (51%) Black/Afro 39 (13%) Hispanos 59 (20%) Other 27 (9%) Asian/ Pacific islanders 18 (6%) American Indians 3 (1%)	Lesbians 256 (86.2%) Bisexual women 41 (13.8%)
Merrill & Wolfe. [38]	Quantitative	USA	White E/C 15 (29%) Black/Afro 15 (29%) Hispanos 10 (19%) Others 4 (7%) American Indians 2 (4%)	Gays 50 (96%) Bisexual men 2 (4%)
Saldivia et al. [39]	Quantitative	Chile	Chile 631 (100%)	Men 222 (35.2%) Women 409 (64.8%)
Toro-Alfonso & Rodríguez-Madera. [40]	Quantitative	Puerto Rico	Puerto Rico 200 (100%)	Gays 165 (83%) Bisexual men 35 (17%)
Islam. [41]	Quantitative	USA	White E/C 126 (68.9%) Black/Afro 20 (10.9%) Hispanos 28 (15.3%) Other non-Hispanic 8 (4.4%)	Lesbians 79 (43.1%) Bisexual women 104 (56.9%)
Franco. [42]	Qualitative	Chile	Chile 20 (100%)	Gays 20 (100%)
Kubicek et al. [43]	Qualitative	USA	White E/C 15 (15%) Black/Afro 25 (25%) Hispanos 35 (35%) Asian/ Pacific islanders 7 (7%) Multiethnic 19 (19%)	Gays/MSM 72 (72%) Bisexual men 27 (27%)
López & Ayala. [44]	Qualitative	Puerto Rico	Puerto Rico 7 (100%)	Lesbians 6 (85%)

Table 1. Cont.

Article	Method	Country of First Author	Origin of Participants	Sexual Orientation/Sexual Practice
Rondan et al. [45]	Qualitative	Peru	Peru 17 (100%)	Lesbians 3 (17.6%) Gays 8 (47%) Bisexual women 6 (35.3%)
Ronzón-Tirado et al. [46]	Qualitative	Mexico	Mexico 15 (100%)	Gays 8 (53.3%) Lesbians 6 (40%) Bisexual woman 1 (6.6%)
Téllez-Santaya & Walters. [47]	Mixed method	Spain	Cuba 70 (100%)	Homosexuals 70 (100%)

Note: White E/C: White European/Caucasian; Black/Afro: Black/Afro-Americans.

In order to ascertain both the study's origin and participant demographics, we considered the country of the institution to be affiliated with the first author for the former aspect. In the latter case, classification was established according to the participants' country or place of origin. It was noted that nine of the investigations came from the United States [26,30,31,33,34,37,38,41,43], four of them from Chile [25,35,39,42], four from Puerto Rico [32,36,40,44], two from Spain [29,47], two from Mexico [27,46], one from Colombia [28] and one from Peru [45].

Regarding the origin of the participants, there was a diversity. In the nine studies conducted in the United States, the presence of Hispanic American participants was limited, with an average of 22.1% not specifying their nationalities. In the two studies conducted in Spain, a total of 68.5% of Hispanic-American participants from countries such as Mexico, Venezuela, Chile, and Cuba were included. In addition, the 12 studies conducted in Hispanic America had a 100% participation of individuals from countries such as Puerto Rico, Mexico, Chile, Peru, and Colombia.

As for the sexual orientation of the participants in the selected studies, the participation of gay individuals was predominant over other sexual orientations, such as lesbians, bisexual men, bisexual women, and pansexual.

As far as gender identity is concerned, there is a predominance of studies conducted on men only [26,27,30,31,33,34,36,38,40,42,43,47]. Secondly, there is research that includes participants of both sexes in the same study [25,28,29,32,35,39,45,46]. Finally, studies conducted only on women are very scarce, with only three identified [37,41,44].

3.2. Risk Factors

The studies analyzed several factors to explain IPV in intragender couples. To describe them, they were organized according to the four levels of the ecological model [14]. Since we intended to study the frequency of risk factors in women, we paid special attention to the results of this population.

3.2.1. Macro-Social System Level

Regarding the macro level, important risk factors related to power dynamics, minority stress in IPV, and education were identified (Table 2).

Table 2. Risk factors: Macro-social system, exosystem and mesosystem variables.

Source	Goal	Power Relationships	Stress of Minorities	Professional Training	Social Support
[29]	To study the influence of insecure attachment style on the perpetration of psychological abuse in same-sex couples, and the moderating role of the level of externality as an antecedent variable of psychological abuse perpetration.	Lack of power and control is reacted to with high levels of insecure attachment.	Outness is linked to social support and the absence of social support can act as a stressor.	Not applicable	Lack of social support can act as a stress factor.
[32]	To analyze the expressions of domestic violence in the lesbian, bisexual and transgender homosexual population (LGBT) in Puerto Rico.	Not applicable	Homosexual men deny or minimize violence because of social stigma.	Promote awareness in services to avoid homophobic and lesbophobic reactions	Not applicable
[35]	To describe the experiences of partner violence (PV) in a sample of gay and lesbian women.	Not applicable	Not applicable	Heteronormative laws that do not adequately consider these cases.	Not applicable
[37]	Exploring the idea that the lesbian community may not be conceptualizing violence in lesbian relationships as domestic violence.	Makes use of homophobia and coming out to maintain power and control.	Minority stress intersects with support networks, as the aggressor isolates from their networks and also threatens with outness	The importance of training, research, and community practices in social assistance institutions to address violence in same-sex couples	Minority stress-related support
[39]	To characterize the type of violence in young same-sex couples in Chile during 2016.	Not applicable	Internalized heterosexism leads to rejection of oneself and one's partner.	Not applicable	Not applicable
[41]	To examine perceptions of psychological IPV, sexual minority stigma, and childhood exposure to domestic violence among sexual minority women residing in the US.	Not applicable	Internalized stigma correlates significantly to women's psychological IPV.	Not applicable	An important aspect to break out of violence.

Table 2. Cont.

Source	Goal	Power Relationships	Stress of Minorities	Professional Training	Social Support
[44]	To explore the experiences of domestic violence in a group of lesbian women in Puerto Rico, and to identify the obstacles and facilitators in their processes of help and support as victims of this problem.	Not applicable	Internalized oppression arises from external prejudices and stereotypes.	Lack of interest in training due to homophobia	Uses the isolation of the victim from her support networks as a control mechanism. At the social level there are no support networks due to exclusion and marginalization by government policies.
[45]	To analyze the perceptions of intimate partner violence (IPV) among lesbians, gays and bisexuals (LGB) in metropolitan Lima.	Power is linked to the control produced by jealousy based on emotional insecurity.	Emotional insecurity due to the lack of acceptance of other orientations, which implies not making oneself visible for fear of the consequences.	Not applicable	Social support is not felt due to homophobia or continued isolation from the partner.
[46]	Describing the elements associated with violence in gay and lesbian relationships.	A means to solve conflicts	Outness triggered the rupture of close ties, generating a progressive isolation so that the only person it contains is the partner.	Questioning heteronormative models in campaigns related to partner violence	The loss of informal support was influenced by coming out of the closet.

Note: This table exclusively incorporates studies that furnish data concerning the variables outlined within.

Power relations as a risk factor for IPV were addressed by eight studies [26,29,37,43–47], five of which included female participants [29,37,44–46]. A relationship was found between individual variables, such as an insecure attachment style [29]. It was identified that a mechanism of power and control was the use of social homophobia, especially when the victim had not revealed his or her sexual orientation or experienced rejection by friends and family due to his or her sexual orientation and/or practice. Exposing sexual orientation becomes a control tactic [37]. Jealousy also arises as an expression of power imbalance, producing distrust and coercive behaviors of control, which results in feelings of loneliness in the victim [45].

Minority stress was addressed by eleven studies [29,33,34,37,39,41,43–47], seven of which included female participants [29,37,39,41,44–46]. Specifically, the literature examined internalized stigma [39,41,44], outness [29,37,45,46], and external stigma [41,45]. A significant correlation was found between internalized stigma and psychological violence in women [41]. A qualitative study highlighted internalized oppression as a result of prejudice and stereotypes, which can lead people to believe negative or incorrect messages coming from dominant sectors [44].

Outness, it was observed in one study, may act as a risk factor for intragender violence [29]. Another study revealed that the level of outness has a mitigating effect on the relationship between insecure attachment style and the perpetration of psychological abuse [29]. It has been pointed out that not coming out of the closet can be used as a threat to control the partner [37]. Likewise, coming out can result in the breakdown of family ties and gradual isolation from friendships, which is considered a psychosocial risk factor [46].

External stigma was also addressed, which also converged with outness in the emotional insecurity that can arise when disclosing sexual orientation or practice to society, which might influence the decision not to denounce due to fear of facing discrimination [45]. Another study revealed a lack of correlation between external stigma and the perception of psychological violence in same-sex couples, suggesting the existence of differences in behaviors and perceptions that require further exploration [45].

Regarding education, five studies addressed the issue as a possible risk factor [25,28,32,33,35], four of which included female participants [25,28,32,35]. One of the latter studies indicated that the higher the level of education, the lower the probability of victimization [35]. However, other studies reported no significant association between education and violence [25,28,32].

3.2.2. Exosystem Level

We identified problems in the exosystem in relation to the preparation of professionals who directly intervene in cases (police and health professionals), as well as in the way the media address this issue. Ten studies [32–35,37,40,42–44,46] problematized this situation, five of which included the participation of women [32,35,37,44,46]. These studies pointed to the need to train professionals on violence in same-sex couples, but a lack of interest has been noted due to homophobia [44]. Training, research, and community-based practices in social support institutions can help lesbians obtain information to compare the cycle of violence in heterosexual and battered lesbian relationships [37].

Other studies problematize the legal regulations, which, in cases of domestic violence, are heteronormative; therefore, it is necessary to have specific regulations to intervene in intra-family violence [35,44].

The media show heteronormative models in campaigns on violence, which generates alienation in this population because they do not feel represented [46].

3.2.3. Mesosystem Level

The mesosystem refers to instrumental or emotional support from the environment [48]. It was addressed by eleven studies [28,29,34,37,38,41–46], seven of which included female participants [28,29,37,41,44–46]. These studies problematized social support as a risk factor in intragender violence because the lack of support, whether informal, formal or the perception of its non-existence limits the possibility of seeking help. In the case of informal social support, this comes mainly from friends and relatives but may be diminished or nullified due to the actions of the aggressor [37,44], especially due to the lack of trust in the family environment, influenced by the process of disclosing their sexual orientation and the consequent fear of discrimination [29,46].

In the case of a lack of formal support (laws and public policies), some studies indicate that it acts as a limiting factor when seeking help [28,44], which in some cases contributes to staying in a violent relationship. In the context of violence among women, social support in general was identified as a key element when breaking out of situations of violence [41].

3.2.4. Micro-System Level

From the microsystem, studies addressed risk factors such as substance use (alcohol or other drugs), mental health, specifically depression, age, and a history of violence and sexual abuse in childhood. Finally, from a relational perspective, sexually transmitted diseases were also included (Table 3).

Table 3. Risk factors: Micro-system variables.

Source	HIV or STI	Substance Consumption	Depression/ Suicidal Ideas	Sociodemographic Factors
[25]	Not applicable	In gay victims of violence, alcohol consumption is higher. No differences were found in lesbians. Consumption of other substances was not significant.	Variable suicidal ideation was not significant between victims and non-victims. Not relevant in lesbians	There are no significant differences in age and professional status between gay victims and non-victims.
[28]	Not applicable	Not applicable	Not applicable	There are no significant differences in sociodemographic variables and IPV
[32]	Not applicable	Consumption of alcohol and other substances in IPV episodes was higher in lesbians.	Not applicable	Education is not significantly related to IPV.
[35]	Not applicable	Not applicable	Not applicable	More education, less victimization.
[39]	HIV is not recognized as a problem in female-to-female relationships.	Not applicable	Not applicable	Not applicable
[43]	Not applicable	Alcohol present in childhood violence, drinking father and aggressor. Within the couple, it was present in episodes of IPV	Not applicable	Not applicable

Note: This table exclusively incorporates studies that furnish data concerning the variables outlined within.

With respect to alcohol and/or drug use, of the eleven studies that addressed this issue [25–27,30,32,34,36,40,43,44,47], four involved women [25,27,32,44]. No significant differences were found between alcohol or drug use and violence in lesbian couples [25,32]. In another study, the consumption of alcohol or other drugs was present as a risk factor in some episodes of violence, and consumption was a behavior learned since childhood [44].

Regarding the exclusive use of other substances, a study that included women reported that drug use could be related to the transmission of HIV [27], but it does not explain differences with other sexual orientations.

Concerning depression, seven studies addressed this [26,30,31,34,40,47], none of which included female participants in their studies. One study in the male population referred to depression as an indirect risk factor for violence [26], while others identified it as an effect of violence.

Another individual risk factor observed in these studies was age. This variable was analyzed by four studies [25,26,28,31], two of which included the participation of women [25,28]. These studies found no significant associations with violence in research involving female participants.

In the family setting, a childhood history of violence and child sexual abuse were addressed. Seven studies addressed childhood violence [26,36,40,41,44,46,47], of which three included female participants [41,44,46]. The results indicated that childhood exposure to models of violent behavior in families played an important role in the learning of behavioral patterns that could affect intimate relationships. According to a study, the degree of exposure to violence could act as an additive factor in situations of violence in female couples, as well as increasing tolerance to psychological violence [41]. This history of violence against women can leave a lasting impact, generating feelings of fear, insecurity, and frustration [44].

In the case of child sexual abuse, this was addressed in only three studies, which included only male participants [26,40,47]. However, no significant association was found between child sexual abuse in men and violence within relationships. It is important to note that this aspect was not problematized in any study that included women.

Among the risk factors in relationships, the presence of sexually transmitted infections (STIs) was noteworthy, with HIV being the most studied in this context. However, it was mainly problematized as a form of intimate partner violence in the male population, according to several studies [27,30,31,33,34,36,39,40,43]. It is worth mentioning that, despite the inclusion of two studies with female participants, this topic was not addressed in a significant way [27,39].

4. Discussion

This scoping review had two goals: to contextualize the prevalence of studies involving female-to-female IPV in comparison to other intragender relationships in Hispanic American while also focusing on identifying the main associated risk factors.

Below, we discuss the incidence of studies on relationships between women, including sexual orientations and practices, study sources, and participants. In addition, the main associated risk factors are described. For the latter, the ecological model [14] was used to organize risk factors, which allowed for a broader understanding of violence from an environmental and contextual perspective.

The volume of studies on IPV in women to date is scarce [3,49]: an aspect that can be confirmed in the current review. The reviewed publications are dominated by studies focusing on male couples compared to female couples. This situation can lead to an overrepresentation of the needs of some groups (gays in this case) compared to others, making the reality of IPV among female couples invisible. Second, this disproportionality of the studies may tend to perpetuate the stereotypical directionality of violence depending on the gender of the aggressor [50,51]. As a result, there is a persisting misconception that violence within female couples is rare or isolated.

Research on sexual orientations and practices in women shows an imbalance, with more attention on lesbians than on bisexual women [22], pansexual, and other sexual orientations/practices. This could generate reductionist assumptions that automatically consider all women in affective–sexual relationships with other women as lesbians. Some studies indicate that bisexual women are more likely to experience violence compared to lesbians [3,9], although little research has been conducted in this area. It is essential to study and consider different sexual orientations and practices to understand the specific risk factors that might be affecting them.

Regarding sexual practices, studies predominantly categorize MSM, but in no case do they use the concept of women who have sex with women (WSW). This may suggest that there are still many taboos in the research regarding gender roles and how women experience their sexuality, which could also influence how sexual violence among women is viewed.

The presence of Hispanic American studies and participants in research on this topic is limited. Most of the studies originate in the U.S., and the participation of Hispanic American individuals is scarce. In addition, there is a lack of representation of several Hispanic American nationalities, among them: Argentina, Paraguay, Uruguay, Bolivia, Ecuador, and the rest of the Central American countries. This points to the need for further research on this issue in this specific context [52].

In relation to risk factors, the ecological model provided an integrative understanding of the various factors involved in IPV among women, as well as an understanding of the interrelationship between the different factors.

Among the risk factors identified in the macrosystem, power relations, minority stress, and education were identified. Power relations influenced and interacted with other factors. However, the main challenge resides in understanding how, up until now, power has been explained based on heteronormative models, where gender plays a fundamental role in its attribution, which is not applicable to intragender violence. Therefore, in order to understand the power dynamics in women's couple relationships, it is necessary to consider gender stereotypes [53–55], which portray, for example, women as harmless, non-violent, and physically weak [56].

Regarding minority stress, known as identity abuse (IA) [9,19,20,49], in the context of intragender violence, the reviewed studies have identified internalized and externalized stigma as major factors in relation to the disclosure of the partner's sexual orientation, known as outness, as a tactic of control and threat. This leads to a gradual decrease in nearby support networks [9,19,20,49]. In addition, it was observed that outness not only affects the close environment but also the search for help in institutions, which links it closely to the mesosystem and support networks.

Even though the problematization of specific factors of IPV in intragender couples, and especially in women, is an advance, what was found in the Hispanic American population and the context investigated is not enough since other studies have delved even deeper into this issue and found other tactics of identity abuse. These consist of undermining, attacking, or denying the partner's identity as a member of the LGTBIQ+ community [9,20,57], as well as the use of derogatory language regarding their sexual orientation [20,57]. These tactics were not detected in the selected studies.

Finally, regarding the education variable, there are discrepancies among studies. One of them suggested that there was no association between violence and education, while another stated quite the opposite. This last statement is in line with other studies conducted in heterosexual populations, which found that as women gain access to political and social rights, as well as to education and employment, their independence increases, which gives them a greater chance of escaping violence [58,59]. Therefore, it is necessary to further study its association with IPV in female couples.

In relation to the exosystem, the importance of this lies in the identification of the multiple indirect effects of violence that have been traditionally ignored [60]. Some research has suggested the need for education and training programs on same-sex partner violence for service providers who are not prepared to serve LGBT people, such as health, social services, and criminal justice professionals [49,61,62]. This awareness is important for reducing behaviors that perpetuate stereotypes and patterns of discrimination against LGBTQ people [3,63] and, specifically, for relationships between women. The scarcity of studies that problematize the impact of the media in the construction of violence and its lack of training on sexual diversity issues is noteworthy.

In the mesosystem, support networks and the IA are closely related. Social support is crucial for breaking out of situations of violence, and a lack of this support is considered an important risk factor in intragender couples, as affected individuals are often isolated from their environment. Some studies have indicated that isolation from external communities of support, such as LGTBIQ+, can be especially harmful to non-heterosexual and non-cisgender survivors. This is because, upon the disclosure of their sexual orientation or gender identity, they often lose the support of their family networks; therefore, this community becomes one of the few support networks that is left for them [20,64]. It is important to consider that cultural values among Latinx individuals, such as "familismo", which often results in prioritizing family connections and collective welfare over personal wants and needs, are linked to a diverse range of family reactions toward sexual minorities [65]. Healthcare professionals should consider the diverse manners through which cultural elements might impact how families respond to individuals identifying as sexual minorities.

The lack of formal support in terms of public policies is a recurring issue, which is reflected in the absence of legislation and adequate training for health professionals and security forces in relation to intragender violence in female couples. This is due, in part, to the predominant conception of violence as a heterosexual phenomenon with a male aggressor and a female victim. In addition, when seeking help, victims face stigma, which generates shame when acknowledging the facts and fears that their accusations will not be taken seriously [22,66,67]. This is an issue that has been scarcely problematized in Hispanic American studies, but it is fundamental to developing strategies that can support both the victims and the perpetrators of violence.

At the microsystem level, risk factors such as alcohol and/or substance use and mental health (depression) and family factors such as childhood violence and child sexual abuse were identified. Finally, at the relational level, STDs were also identified.

Regarding alcohol consumption, it is believed that high consumption may be associated with an elevated rate of intimate partner violence in female couples [67,68], although there are few studies that support this association [68]. It has been observed that alcoholism can be a risk factor contributing to episodes of violence when combined with other macrosystemic and microsystemic determinants, which does not imply that alcohol abuse and/or dependence are a cause of violence [69].

According to some studies, it has been observed that depression might be present in cases of domestic violence, but it is considered more as an effect of violence itself [70]. In addition, a relationship has been established between depression and other factors, such as post-traumatic stress [71].

In short, there were discrepancies in the studies on alcohol consumption and depression due to their possible relationship as a cause and consequence of violence, which suggests the need for further research on these topics.

With regard to experiences of violence in childhood, studies have found links with abusive relationships in adulthood [72]. Some studies suggest that violence in childhood may have an additive effect on the likelihood of becoming involved in violent relationships in adulthood [4], generating fear and insecurity in those who have experienced violence. However, there are discrepancies as to the strength and straightforwardness of this association [72,73].

Childhood sexual abuse was not addressed by studies that included women, only in those that included men. In the latter, it was not significantly associated with or predictive of IPV.

Finally, the relationship between HIV and IPV has been studied mainly in heterosexual couples and male couples, with inconclusive results in female couples. However, IPV has been found to increase the risk of HIV infection and may lead to the victimization of HIV-positive individuals [74,75]. The sexual coercion that leads to exposure to HIV is recognized as violence within a relationship [76]. The lack of recognition of this problem in women involved in emotional and sexual relationships with other women makes them especially vulnerable since they are invisible in preventive campaigns. The mistaken beliefs about female sexuality and its associated risks complicate this situation even more since it can be used as a form of violence without being aware of it. Therefore, the lack of existing education that problematizes these aspects is also a risk factor.

Limitations

This scoping review comes with some limitations. First, to include studies made only in English and Spanish means we excluded attention to research made in other languages. Second, the low number of investigations found in couples of women in a Hispanic-American context could compromise the results and their external validity. Third, the low number of studies that use qualitative and/or mixed methods, together with the low representativeness of participants of diverse sexual orientations, could make it difficult to understand the phenomenon and its risk factors.

5. Conclusions

This scoping review has made it possible to describe the IPV phenomenon in relationships between women in Hispanic America, as well as to identify its risk factors. It is critical to address these factors globally and not individually, as IPV is influenced by a combination of various factors that converge at different points. For instance, the social support and stress experienced by sexual minorities are key elements, as support, both formal and informal, often depends on the acceptance of the existing sexual orientation. To explain the risk factors of IPV among women, it is necessary to problematize and incorporate specific elements of this population, such as identity abuse.

In addition, it is important to consider that, to advance in the investigation of IPV in female couples, it is necessary to question several paradigms in the explanation of violence. Among them is the gender approach, which is insufficient to fully understand violence in this context. However, in future studies, it would be desirable to include research in other languages, as well as to expand the number of investigations focusing on violence in couples of women. This approach should also take into account the diversity of couples within these relationships.

Finally, it is crucial to make this problem visible throughout Latin America since there was a lack of representation of certain nationalities among the participants. It would be desirable to increase the number of studies that use qualitative and/or mixed methods, as well as to achieve a greater representation of different sexual orientations. This shows the need to make visible and address this issue not only at the research level but also in the field of public policies, and therefore, to implement education in healthy relationships and the psychological interventions appropriate to their needs.

Author Contributions: Conceptualization, L.G.-V.; Methodology, L.G.-V., and A.C.-T.; Formal analysis, L.G.-V., A.C.-T. and I.A.-T.; Data curation, L.G.-V.; Writing—original draft preparation, L.G.-V.; Writing—review and editing, L.G.-V., A.C.-T. and I.A.-T.; Supervision, A.C.-T. and I.A.-T. All authors have read and agreed to the published version of the manuscript.

Funding: This research was funded by CONICYT, grant number "72200443" and by the "Research Group in Social, Environmental and Organizational Psychology, University of Barcelona (PsicoSAO)".

Institutional Review Board Statement: Not applicable.

Informed Consent Statement: Not applicable.

Data Availability Statement: Not applicable.

Conflicts of Interest: The authors declare no conflict of interest.

References

1. Walters, L.; Chen, J.; Breiding, M. *The National Intimate Partner and Sexual Violence Survey (NISVS): 2010 Findings on Victimization by Sexual Orientation*; National Center for Injury Prevention and Control, Centers for Disease Control and Prevention: Atlanta, GA, USA, 2013.
2. Breiding, M.; Basile, K.; Smith, S.; Black, M.; Mahendra, R. *Intimate Partner Violence Surveillance Uniform Definitions and Recommended Data Elements, Version 2.0*; National Center for Injury Prevention and Control, Centers for Disease Control and Prevention: Atlanta, GA, USA, 2015.
3. Longobardi, C.; Badenes-Ribera, L. Intimate Partner Violence in Same-Sex Relationships and The Role of Sexual Minority Stressors: A Systematic Review of the Past 10 Years. *J. Child Fam. Stud.* **2017**, *26*, 2039–2049. [CrossRef]
4. Lagdon, S.; Armour, C.; Stringer, M. Adult experience of mental health outcomes as a result of intimate partner violence victimisation: A systematic review. *Eur. J. Psychotraumatol.* **2014**, *5*, 24794. [CrossRef]
5. Ristock, J.L. *No More Secrets. Violence in Lesbian Relationships*; Routledge: New York, NY, USA, 2002; pp. 1–23.
6. Stiles-Shields, C.; Carroll, R.A. Same-Sex Domestic Violence: Prevalence, Unique Aspects, and Clinical Implications. *J. Sex Marital Ther.* **2015**, *41*, 636–648. [CrossRef]
7. Edwards, K.M.; Sylaska, K.M. Reactions to Participating in Intimate Partner Violence and Minority Stress Research: A Mixed Methodological Study of Self-Identified Lesbian and Gay Emerging Adults. *J. Sex Res.* **2015**, *53*, 655–665. [CrossRef] [PubMed]
8. Langenderfer-Magruder, L.; Whitfield, D.L.; Walls, N.E.; Kattari, S.K.; Ramos, D. Experiences of Intimate Partner Violence and Subsequent Police Reporting Among Lesbian, Gay, Bisexual, Transgender, and Queer Adults in Colorado: Comparing Rates of Cisgender and Transgender Victimization. *J. Interpers. Violence* **2016**, *31*, 855–871. [CrossRef] [PubMed]
9. Balsam, K.F.; Szymanski, D.M. Relationship quality and domestic violence in women's same-sex relationships: The role of minority stress. *Psychol. Women Q.* **2005**, *29*, 258–269. [CrossRef]
10. Sanger, N.; Lynch, I. 'You have to bow right here': Heteronormative scripts and intimate partner violence in women's same-sex relationships. *Cult. Health Sex.* **2017**, *20*, 201–217. [CrossRef]
11. Swan, L.; Henry, R.; Smith, E.; Aguayo, A.; Viridiana, B.; Barajas, R.; Perrin, P. Discrimination and Intimate Partner Violence Victimization and Perpetration Among a Convenience Sample of LGBT Individuals in Latin America. *J. Interpers. Violence* **2019**, *36*, NP8520–NP8537. [CrossRef]
12. Trombetta, T.; Rollè, L. Intimate Partner Violence Perpetration Among Sexual Minority People and Associated Factors: A Systematic Review of Quantitative Studies. *Sex. Res. Soc. Policy* **2023**, *20*, 886–935. [CrossRef]
13. Pita, S.; Vila, M.; Carpente, J. Determinación de factores de riesgo Pita. *Cad. Atención Primaria* **2002**, *48*, 75–78.
14. Bronfenbrenner, U. *La Ecologia del Desarrollo Humano. Experimentos en Entornos Naturales y Diseñados*; Paidós Ibérica: Barcelona, Spain, 1987; pp. 231–281.
15. Frías, S.M. Ámbitos y formas de violencia contra mujeres y niñas: Evidencias a partir de las encuestas. *Acta Sociol.* **2014**, *65*, 11–36. [CrossRef]
16. Meyer, I.H. Prejudice, Social Stress, and Mental Health in Lesbian, Gay, and Bisexual Populations: Conceptual Issues and Research Evidence. *Psychol. Bull.* **2003**, *129*, 674–697. [CrossRef]
17. Reyes, M.; Alday, A.; Aurellano, A.; Escala, S.; Hernandez, P.; Matienzo, J.; Panaguiton, K.; Tan, A.; Zsila, A. Minority Stressors and Attitudes Toward Intimate Partner Violence among Lesbian and Gay Individuals. *Sex. Cult.* **2023**, *27*, 930–950. [CrossRef]
18. Balik, C.; Bilgin, H. Experiences of Minority Stress and Intimate Partner Violence Among Homosexual Women in Turkey. *J. Interpers. Violence* **2019**, *36*, 8984–9007. [CrossRef] [PubMed]
19. Ard, K.L.; Makadon, H.J. Addressing intimate partner violence in lesbian, gay, bisexual, and transgender patients. *J. Gen. Intern. Med.* **2011**, *26*, 930–933. [CrossRef]
20. Woulfe, J.M.; Goodman, L.A. Identity Abuse as a Tactic of Violence in LGBTQ Communities: Initial Validation of the Identity Abuse Measure. *J. Interpers. Violence* **2018**, *36*, 2656–2676. [CrossRef] [PubMed]
21. Tricco, A.C.; Lillie, E.; Zarin, W.; O'Brien, K.K.; Colquhoun, H.; Levac, D.; Moher, D.; Peters, M.D.J.; Horsley, T.; Weeks, L.; et al. PRISMA extension for scoping reviews (PRISMA-ScR): Checklist and explanation. *Ann. Intern. Med.* **2018**, *169*, 467–473. [CrossRef]
22. Peterson, C.H.; Peterson, N.A.; Cheng, Y.-J.; Dalley, L.M.; Flowers, K.M. A Systematic Review of Standardized Assessments of Couple and Family Constructs in GLBT Populations. *J. GLBT Fam. Stud.* **2020**, *16*, 455–474. [CrossRef]
23. Munn, Z.; Peters, M.D.J.; Stern, C.; Tufanaru, C.; McArthur, A.; Aromataris, E. Systematic review or scoping review? Guidance for authors when choosing between a systematic or scoping review approach. *BMC Med. Res. Methodol.* **2018**, *18*, 143. [CrossRef] [PubMed]
24. Braun, V.; Clarke, V. Using thematic analysis in psychology, Qualitative Research in Psychology. *Qual. Res. Psychol.* **2006**, *3*, 77–101. [CrossRef]
25. Barrientos, J.; Escartín, J.; Longares, L.; Rodríguez-Carballeira, Á. Sociodemographic characteristics of gay and lesbian victims of intimate partner psychological abuse in Spain and Latin America/Características sociodemográficas de gais y lesbianas víctimas de abuso psicológico en pareja en España e Hispanoamérica. *Rev. Psicol. Soc.* **2018**, *33*, 240–274. [CrossRef]
26. Bosco, S.C.; Robles, G.; Stephenson, R.; Starks, T.J. Relationship Power and Intimate Partner Violence in Sexual Minority Male Couples. *J. Interpers. Violence* **2020**, *37*, NP671–NP695. [CrossRef]

27. Rodríguez, L.; Lara, M. HIV as a means of materializing Gender Violence and violence in same-sex couples. *Enferm. Glob.* **2021**, *62*, 196–215. [CrossRef]
28. Redondo-Pacheco, J.; Rey-García, P.; Ibarra-Mojica, A.; Luzardo-Briceño, M. Violencia intragénero entre parejas homosexuales en universitarios de Bucaramanga, Colombia. *Univ. y Salud* **2021**, *23*, 217–227. [CrossRef]
29. Longares, L.; Escartín, J.; Barrientos, J.; Rodríguez-Carballeira, Á. Insecure Attachment and Perpetration of Psychological Abuse in Same-Sex Couples: A Relationship Moderated by Outness. *Sex. Res. Soc. Policy* **2018**, *17*, 1–12. [CrossRef]
30. Davis, A.; Kaighobadi, F.; Stephenson, R.; Rael, C.; Sandfort, T. Associations between Alcohol Use and Intimate Partner Violence among Men Who Have Sex with Men. *LGBT Health* **2016**, *3*, 400–406. [CrossRef]
31. Stephenson, R.; Khosropour, C.; Sullivan, P. Reporting of Intimate Partner Violence among Men Who Have Sex with Men in an Online Survey. *West. J. Emerg. Med.* **2010**, *11*, 242–246. [PubMed]
32. Reyes, F.; Rodríguez, J.R.; Malavé, S. Manifestaciones de la violencia doméstica en una muestra de hombres homosexuales y mujeres lesbianas puertorriqueñas. *Interam. J. Psychol.* **2005**, *39*, 449–456.
33. Loveland, J.E.; Raghavan, C. Near-Lethal Violence in a Sample of High-Risk Men in Same-Sex Relationships. *Psychol. Sex. Orientat. Gend. Divers.* **2014**, *1*, 51–62. [CrossRef]
34. Houston, E.; McKirnan, D.J. Intimate partner abuse among gay and bisexual men: Risk correlates and health outcomes. *J. Urban Health* **2007**, *84*, 681–690. [CrossRef]
35. Gómez, F.; Barrientos Delgado, J.; Guzmán González, M.; Cárdenas Castro, M.; Bahamondes Correa, J. Violencia de pareja en hombres gay y mujeres Lesbianas Chilenas: Un estudio exploratorio. *Interdisciplinaria* **2017**, *34*, 57–72. [CrossRef]
36. Rodríguez, S.; Toro-Alfonso, J. Description of a domestic violence measure for Puerto Rican gay males. *J. Homosex.* **2005**, *50*, 155–173. [CrossRef]
37. McLaughlin, E.M.; Rozee, P.D. Knowledge about heterosexual versus lesbian battering among lesbians. *Intim. Betrayal Domest. Violence Lesbian Relatsh.* **2001**, *23*, 39–58. [CrossRef]
38. Merrill, G.S.; Wolfe, V.A. Battered gay men: An exploration of abuse, help seeking, and why they stay. *J. Homosex.* **2000**, *39*, 1–30. [CrossRef] [PubMed]
39. Saldivia, C.; Faúndez, B.; Sotomayor, S.; Cea, F. Violencia íntima en parejas jóvenes del mismo sexo en Chile. *Última Década* **2017**, *25*, 184–212. [CrossRef]
40. Toro-Alfonso, J.; Rodríguez-Madera, S. Domestic violence in Puerto Rican gay male couples: Perceived prevalence, intergenerational violence, addictive behaviors, and conflict resolution skills. *J. Interpers. Violence* **2004**, *19*, 639–654. [CrossRef] [PubMed]
41. Islam, S. Perceptions of psychological intimate partner violence: The influence of sexual minority stigma and childhood exposure to domestic violence among bisexual and lesbian women. *Int. J. Environ. Res. Public Health* **2021**, *18*, 5356. [CrossRef]
42. Franco, M.A. Caracterización de las representaciones sociales de la violencia intragénero en parejas de hombres gay. Caso: Ciudad de Temuco-Chile. *Hum. Rev. Int. Humanit. Rev. Rev. Int. Humanidades* **2022**, *11*, 1–9. [CrossRef]
43. Kubicek, K.; McNeeley, M.; Collins, S. "Same-Sex Relationship in a Straight World": Individual and Societal Influences on Power and Control in Young Men's Relationships. *J. Interpers. Violence* **2015**, *30*, 83–109. [CrossRef]
44. López, M.; Ayala, D. Intimidad y las múltiples manifestaciones de la violencia doméstica entre mujeres lesbianas. *Salud Soc.* **2011**, *2*, 151–174. [CrossRef]
45. Rondan, L.-B.; Rojas, S.; Cruz-Manrique, Y.R.; Malvaceda-Espinoza, E.L. Violencia Íntima de Pareja, en parejas lesbianas, gais y bisexuales de Lima Metropolitana. *Rev. Investig. Psicol.* **2022**, *25*, 105–120. [CrossRef]
46. Ronzón-Tirado, R.C.; Rey, L.; del Pilar González-Flores, M. Modelos parentales y su relación con la violencia en las parejas del mismo sexo. *Rev. Latinoam. Cienc. Soc. Niñez Juv.* **2017**, *15*, 1137–1147. [CrossRef]
47. Téllez-Santaya, P.; Walters, A.S. Intimate Partner Violence Within Gay Male Couples: Dimensionalizing Partner Violence Among Cuban Gay Men. *Sex. Cult.* **2011**, *15*, 153–178. [CrossRef]
48. Rivas, E.; Panadero, S.; Bonilla, E.; Vásquez, R.; Vázquez, J.J. Influencia del apoyo social en el mantenimiento de la convivencia con el agresor en víctimas de violencia de género de León (Nicaragua). *Inf. Psicol.* **2018**, *18*, 145–165. [CrossRef]
49. West, C.M. Lesbian intimate partner violence: Prevalence and dynamics. *J. Lesbian Stud.* **2002**, *6*, 121–127. [CrossRef]
50. Cantera, L. Aproximación empírica a la agenda oculta en el campo de la violencia en la pareja. *Psychosoc. Interv.* **2004**, *13*, 219–230.
51. Cantera, L.; Gamero, V. La violencia en la pareja a la luz de los estereotipos de género. *Psico* **2007**, *38*, 233–237.
52. Barrientos, J.; Rodríguez Carballeira, Á.; Escartín Solanelles, J.; Longares, L. Violencia en parejas del mismo sexo:revisión y perspectivas actuales/Intimate same-sex partner violence: Review and outlook. *Rev. Argent. Clínica Psicol.* **2016**, *XXV*, 289–298.
53. Rollè, L.; Giardina, G.; Caldarera, A.M.; Gerino, E.; Brustia, P. When intimate partner violence meets same sex couples: A review of same sex intimate partner violence. *Front. Psychol.* **2018**, *9*, 1506. [CrossRef]
54. Brown, C. Gender-role implications on same-sex intimate partner abuse. *J. Fam. Violence* **2008**, *23*, 457–462. [CrossRef]
55. Little, B.; Terrance, C. Perceptions of domestic violence in lesbian relationships: Stereotypes and gender role expectations. *J. Homosex.* **2010**, *57*, 429–440. [CrossRef] [PubMed]
56. Ristock, J.L. *Relationship Violence in Lesbian/Gay/Bisexual/Transgender/Queer [LGBTQ] Communities Moving Beyond a Gender-Based Framework*; Violence Against Women Online Resources: Harrisburg, PA, USA, 2005; pp. 1–19. Available online: http://www.mincava.umn.edu/documents/lgbtqviolence/lgbtqviolence.pdf (accessed on 17 March 2023).

57. National Center on Domestic & Sexual Violence. *Gay, Lesbian, Bisexual, and Trans Power and Control Wheel*; National Center on Domestic and Sexual Violence: Austin, TX, USA, 2014. Available online: http://www.ncdsv.org/images/%0ATCFV_glbt_wheel.pdf (accessed on 17 March 2023).
58. Villarreal, A. Women's Employment Status, Coercive Control, and Intimate Partner Violence in Mexico. *J. Marriage Fam.* **2007**, *69*, 418–434. [CrossRef]
59. Puentes-Martinez, A.; Ubillos-Landa, S.; Echeburúa, E.; Páez-Rovira, D. Factores de riesgo asociados a la violencia sufrida por la mujer en la pareja: Una revisión de meta-análisis y estudios recientes. *Ann. Psychol.* **2016**, *32*, 295–306. [CrossRef]
60. Herrero, J. La perspectiva ecológica. In *Introducción a la Psicología Comunitaria*; Editorial Paidós: Buenos Aires, Argentina, 2004; pp. 99–134.
61. Badenes-Ribera, L.; Bonilla-Campos, A.; Frias-Navarro, D.; Pons-Salvador, G.; Monterde-i-Bort, H. Intimate partner violence in self-identified lesbians: A systematic review of its prevalence and correlates. *Trauma Violence Abus.* **2015**, *17*, 284–297. [CrossRef]
62. Subirana-Malaret, M.; Gahagan, J.; Parker, R. Intersectionality and sex and gender-based analyses as promising approaches in addressing intimate partner violence treatment programs among LGBT couples: A scoping review. *Cogent Soc. Sci.* **2019**, *5*, 1644982. [CrossRef]
63. Messinger, A.M. Bidirectional Same-Gender and Sexual Minority Intimate Partner Violence. *Violence Gend.* **2018**, *5*, 241–249. [CrossRef]
64. Ford, C.L.; Slavin, T.; Hilton, K.L.; Holt, S.L. Intimate Partner Violence Prevention Services and Resources in Los Angeles: Issues, Needs, and Challenges for Assisting Lesbian, Gay, Bisexual, and Transgender Clients. *Health Promot. Pract.* **2013**, *14*, 841–849. [CrossRef] [PubMed]
65. Przeworski, A.; Piedra, A. The Role of the Family for Sexual Minority Latinx Individuals: A Systematic Review and Recommendations for Clinical Practice. *J. GLBT Fam. Stud.* **2020**, *16*, 211–240. [CrossRef]
66. Ristock, J.L. Exploring Dynamics of Abusive Lesbian Relationships: Preliminary Analysis of a Multisite, Qualitative Study. *Am. J. Community Psychol.* **2003**, *31*, 329–341. [CrossRef]
67. Glass, N.; Perrin, N.; Hanson, G.; Bloom, T.; Gardner, E.; Campbell, J.C. Risk for reassault in abusive female same-sex relationships. *Am. J. Public Health* **2008**, *98*, 1021–1027. [CrossRef]
68. Klostermann, K.; Kelley, M.L.; Milletich, R.J.; Mignone, T. Alcoholism and partner aggression among gay and lesbian couples. *Aggress. Violent Behav.* **2011**, *16*, 115–119. [CrossRef]
69. Gil, E.; Lloret, I. La violencia de género. In *Concepto Jurídico de Violencia de Género*; Editorial UOC: Barcelona, Spain, 2007; pp. 41–80.
70. Randle, A.A.; Graham, C.A. A Review of the Evidence on the Effects of Intimate Partner Violence on Men. *Psychol. Men Masculinity* **2011**, *12*, 97–111. [CrossRef]
71. Kessler, R.C.; Molnar, B.E.; Feurer, I.D.; Appelbaum, M. Patterns and mental health predictors of domestic violence in the United States: Results from the National Comorbidity Survey. *Int. J. Law Psychiatry* **2001**, *24*, 487–508. [CrossRef]
72. Smith-Marek, E.N.; Cafferky, B.; Dharnidharka, P.; Mallory, A.B.; Dominguez, M.; High, J.; Stith, S.M.; Mendez, M. Effects of Childhood Experiences of Family Violence on Adult Partner Violence: A Meta-Analytic Review. *J. Fam. Theory Rev.* **2015**, *7*, 498–519. [CrossRef]
73. Haselschwerdt, M.L.; Savasuk-Luxton, R.; Hlavaty, K. A Methodological Review and Critique of the "Intergenerational Transmission of Violence" Literature. *Trauma Violence Abus.* **2019**, *20*, 168–182. [CrossRef] [PubMed]
74. Ramachandran, S.; Yonas, M.A.; Silvestre, A.J.; Burke, J.G. Intimate Partner Violence among HIV Positive Persons in an Urban Clinic. *AIDS Care* **2021**, *22*, 1536–1543. [CrossRef] [PubMed]
75. Carlson, A.; Ghandour, R.M.; Burke, J.G.; Mahoney, P.; McDonnell, K.A.; O'Campo, P. HIV/AIDS and intimate partner violence: Intersecting women's health issues in the United States. *Trauma Violence Abus.* **2008**, *8*, 178–198. [CrossRef]
76. Kalichman, S.; Rompa, D. Sexually coerced and noncoerced gay and bisexual men: Factors relevant to risk for human immunodeficiency virus (HIV) infection. *J. Sex Res.* **1995**, *32*, 45–50. [CrossRef]

Disclaimer/Publisher's Note: The statements, opinions and data contained in all publications are solely those of the individual author(s) and contributor(s) and not of MDPI and/or the editor(s). MDPI and/or the editor(s) disclaim responsibility for any injury to people or property resulting from any ideas, methods, instructions or products referred to in the content.

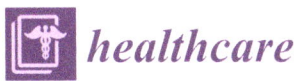

Article

Youth Dating Violence, Behavioral Sensitivity, and Emotional Intelligence: A Mediation Analysis

María Pilar Salguero-Alcañiz [1], Ana Merchán-Clavellino [2,3,*] and Jose Ramón Alameda-Bailén [1,*]

[1] Basic Psychology Area, Department of Clinical and Experimental Psychology, University of Huelva, 21007 Huelva, Spain; pilar.salguero@dpsi.uhu.es
[2] Social Psychology Area, Department of Psychology, University of Cádiz, 11519 Cádiz, Spain
[3] INDESS (Research University Institute for Sustainable Social Development), University of Cádiz, 11406 Jerez de la Frontera, Spain
* Correspondence: ana.merchan@uca.es (A.M.-C.); alameda@uhu.es (J.R.A.-B.)

Abstract: Intimate partner violence is a multidimensional phenomenon encompassing psychological, physical, and sexual components. Violence in young couples is common in our society. This kind of violence is usually bidirectional, which adds to its complexity. This study aimed to explore how victimization (in three dimensions: non-abuse, technical mistreatment, and mistreatment) and perpetration (in two dimensions: non-perpetrator and perpetrator) are related to the BIS (Behavioral Inhibition System)/BAS (Behavioral Approach System), and it also evaluated if the dimensions of emotional intelligence (EI) (emotional attention, clarity, and regulation) mediate this relationship. Violence was evaluated in 272 young volunteer participants, as well as BIS/BAS behavioral sensitivity and perceived emotional intelligence. The correlations between these variables were analyzed, and a mediation analysis was also conducted. The results show that victimization (of the sexual and coercive type) was associated with less BAS activation, while victimization (of the sexual, humiliation, and detachment types) was associated with less BIS activity. All types of victimization were associated with less EI, specifically with less emotional clarity. Aggression (of the sexual, humiliation, detachment, and coercion types) was related to lower BAS and higher BIS sensitivity. Detachment aggression was associated with low emotional clarity. In conclusion, relationships between victimization and perpetration are evidenced in terms of BIS/BAS sensitivity and EI. Specifically, the dimension of EI emotional clarity acts as a mediator of BIS activation in victims of detachment.

Keywords: behavioral sensitivity; emotional intelligence; violence in young couples

Citation: Salguero-Alcañiz, M.P.; Merchán-Clavellino, A.; Alameda-Bailén, J.R. Youth Dating Violence, Behavioral Sensitivity, and Emotional Intelligence: A Mediation Analysis. *Healthcare* **2023**, *11*, 2445. https://doi.org/10.3390/healthcare11172445

Academic Editors: Isabel Cuadrado-Gordillo, Parra Guadalupe Martín-Mora and John H. Foster

Received: 28 July 2023
Revised: 26 August 2023
Accepted: 30 August 2023
Published: 31 August 2023

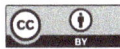

Copyright: © 2023 by the authors. Licensee MDPI, Basel, Switzerland. This article is an open access article distributed under the terms and conditions of the Creative Commons Attribution (CC BY) license (https://creativecommons.org/licenses/by/4.0/).

1. Introduction

Intimate partner violence is a multidimensional phenomenon that encompasses psychological, physical, and sexual components [1], and it can emerge at any time in the relationship. Intimate partner violence is increasingly appearing at younger ages [2] and in both sexes [3].

Violence within couples is a complex issue with various elements that should be considered comprehensively. This phenomenon extends beyond traditional stereotypes of male-perpetrated physical violence, where men are the aggressors and women the victims [4,5]. This approach is reductionist and is not appropriate for addressing a phenomenon as complex and heterogeneous as couple violence. In this paper, we focus on some factors (behavioral sensitivity and emotional intelligence) that may be important but are not the only ones that potentially contribute to dating violence.

Violence in young couples is different from that in adult couples [4]. Recent studies on violence in young couples indicate that both men and women are equally likely to perpetrate violence [6–12]. Thus, both sexes have the same predisposition to perpetrate violence [10]. Recently, Conroy et al. [13] demonstrated that problematic attitudes towards violence are not limited to men but also exist in women. Furthermore, bidirectional violence, where both partners act as both aggressors and victims interchangeably, is currently the most prevalent form [5–8,11,13–19]. This is more pronounced in psychological attacks compared to physical ones [14]. Nevertheless, there are sex differences, as women perpetrate both psychological and physical violence, while physical violence prevails among men [9–11,20–22]. This signals a need to raise awareness of abuse perpetrated by women against men so that they can ask for help without feeling ashamed.

Violence is not a spontaneous or natural phenomenon [5]. Men and women intentionally learn to use violent behaviors to harm their respective partners [23,24]. Therefore, learning plays a crucial role in the emergence and persistence of violent behavior. Violent behavior also has emotional and motivational components, akin to other learned behavior. Additionality, it is essential to not only examine the cognitive and emotional variables associated with the aggressor's profile, as is traditionally done, but also, according to more recent theoretical perspectives, the determinants of the victim's profile [25].

In this context, the theory of behavioral sensitivity [26–28] provides an integrated approach for understanding behavior from a personality perspective, encompassing emotion, motivation, and learning. This theory is based on two complementary behavioral systems: the Behavioral Activation System (BAS) and the Behavioral Inhibition System (BIS). Each system involves different neural correlates specialized in detecting, processing, and responding to certain stimuli [29]. These motivational systems can trigger emotional and behavioral responses in threatening situations [30,31].

The BAS specializes in processing information related to incentives and rewards, leading to positive feelings like hope and euphoria and motivating approach behaviors. Individuals with high BAS sensitivity exhibit this response even to small incentives [32]. Conversely, the BIS system processes information related to punishment, aversive stimuli, and threats, causing arousal and heightened attention to threats when danger signals are present. People with high BIS sensitivity experience distress and anxiety even in response to minimal threats [32].

The relationship between BIS/BAS behavioral sensitivity and intimate partner violence has not been systematically explored. However, Meyer et al. [31] examined the relationship between the BIS/BAS scales and the hypothetical threat of losing a partner, finding significant associations between the activations of both systems (BIS and BAS) and the threat of partner loss. These findings are significant as they reveal a close connection between the threat of partner loss and the different psychological profiles of both victims of abuse and perpetrators of different types of violence.

Hence, the behavioral sensitivity theory [29] highlights the fundamental role that motivations and emotions play in learning. The construct of emotional intelligence (EI) is also relevant in this context as it reflects the inseparable link between cognition and emotion [33]. The most widely accepted definition of EI defines it as "the ability to accurately perceive, assess and express emotions, the ability to access and/or generate feelings that facilitate thought; the ability to understand emotions and emotional knowledge and the ability to regulate emotions promoting emotional and intellectual growth" ([34], p. 5).

The association between EI and violence in young couples has been previously described. García González and Quezada [35] found that EI enhances satisfaction in couple relationships by aiding in the resolution of inherent conflicts, while a low level of EI is associated with stress and violence in relationships. This link between EI and violence has also been emphasized by Zapata [36], showing a significant negative correlation between EI and the dimensions of coercion, physical, detachment, and humiliation perpetration. This aligns with the proposal of Moreno et al. [37], which consists of the implementation of programs based on the acquisition of EI skills to reduce and/or prevent violence in young couples.

Furthermore, various studies have described the association between EI and affective states, indicating that high EI is associated with a positive mood, while low EI is linked to a negative mood [37–40].

The BIS/BAS systems are also related to EI, with high EI being characterized by reward sensitivity (BAS) and low EI being associated with low BIS activation [38]. This relationship between the BIS/BAS systems and EI appears to involve mediation, wherein EI modulates the effects of the BIS/BAS systems on emotions, feelings, and moods.

Hence, it is plausible that both the BIS/BAS systems and EI are variables that play a role in the behavior of couples, both victims and aggressors, who engage in violence.

Therefore, this work aimed to analyze the relationship between the BIS/BAS systems and EI in the violent behavior of young couples, as well as the directionality of this relationship, to understand the risk and vulnerability factors associated with couple violence, both in both victims and aggressors. This understanding can lead to more targeted and effective preventive interventions.

Consequently, the hypothesis of this study posits that both victims and aggressors will score higher on the BIS and lower on the BAS. Additionally, both victims and aggressors are expected to exhibit low levels of EI.

2. Materials and Methods

2.1. Participants

The sample included 272 Spanish volunteer participants, with a mean age of 20.97 years ($SD = 2.52$), ranging from 19 to 30 years old (82.7% women). Approximately half of the participants had studied at the university level (52.2%), 1.8% of them had a master's degree, 33.1% had a bachelor's degree, 12.5% had vocational training, and 0.4% had completed secondary education.

2.2. Procedure

Data were collected using self-administered online questionnaires, using the random sampling method. Participation was anonymous and the data were recorded confidentially. All participants were informed of the study objectives and the possibility of dropping out of the study at any time. The study was conducted according to the 1975 Declaration of Helsinki of the World Medical Association (amended by the 64th General Assembly, Fortaleza, Brazil, October 2013), and all participants signed the written informed consent form.

2.3. Instruments

An ad hoc questionnaire was developed to record the sociodemographic information of the participants. The requested data were sex, age, and current educational level.

Revised Dating Violence Questionnaire (DVQ-R) [40]: This questionnaire evaluates two categories in the evaluation of violence: victimization and perpetration. Scores are obtained on five dimensions for each category: alienation, humiliation, coercion, physical violence, and sexual violence. DVQ-R includes 20 items on a Likert-type scale with five response options, ranging from 0 (never) to 4 (all the time). The internal consistency of this questionnaire for the five scales ranges between 0.64 and 0.74 (Cronbach's alpha, α), and for the total scale, the consistency is $\alpha = 0.85$. The internal consistency found in our sample for the five scales ranged between $\alpha = 0.5$ and 0.7 [40–42]. In addition, the perception of abuse was analyzed through three yes/no questions: Are you or have you been afraid of your partner? Do you feel or have you felt trapped in your relationship? Have you ever felt mistreated in your relationship? An α value of 0.6 was obtained for the three items.

The Sensitivity to Punishment (SP) and Sensitivity to Reward (SR) Questionnaire (SPSRQ; [43]): This is a Spanish version of the measurement of the BIS/BAS systems. SPSRQ consists of 48 dichotomous items (yes–no), and it is divided into two 24-item scales: Sensitivity to Punishment (SP) as a measure of the BIS and Sensitivity to Reward (SR) as a measure of the BAS. The reliability of the scale is adequate, with the SP scale showing an α value of 0.83 and the SR scale showing an α value of 0.76 [44]. In our sample, there was an alpha value of 0.8 for SP and 0.7 for SR.

Trait Meta-Mood Scale, TMMS-24 [45]: This scale includes 24 Likert-type items, ranging from 1 to 5. It is divided into three dimensions of perceived emotional intelligence, each with 8 components: emotional attention (ability to identify one's own emotions and the emotions of others and ability to know how to express emotions), emotional clarity (understanding of emotions), and emotional repair or regulation (ability to manage emotions). The reliability and validity indices reported are adequate [46], and these indices were also adequate in our sample. Reliability in attention was $\alpha = 0.8$, $\alpha = 0.9$ in clarity, and $\alpha = 0.8$ in regulation.

2.4. Statistical Analysis

In the preliminary analyses, descriptive statistics (percentages, means, and standard deviations) were calculated, and mean difference *t*-tests (for the variables with two response alternatives) and analysis of variance (ANOVA), for variables with two or more response options (violence group), were conducted to analyze significant differences. Post hoc tests were performed for respective comparisons. Cohen's d was calculated for standardized mean differences, and based on the values obtained, an effect size of less than 0.2 was considered "small", between 0.5 and 0.8, the effect size was considered "medium", and for any value upwards of 0.8, the effect size was considered "large" [47]. Pearson correlations were calculated between the study variables. The internal consistency of the scales was analyzed using Cronbach's alpha coefficient.

The SPSS 25.0 statistical package was used, and according to the macro Process [48], the mediation analysis was established with a 95% confidence interval and a number of bootstrapping samples of 10,000. The estimates of each analysis were calculated through their respective unstandardized regression coefficients (coeff), their standard errors (SEs), t-values and their significance levels (p), and the different values of the lower limit (LLCI) and upper limit (ULCI) of the confidence interval. The interpretation of significance was performed through the values of each LLCI and ULCI. Therefore, when the number 0 was found between this interval, it confirmed that this particular result was not significant. The serial mediation analysis was conducted using model 6 and analyzed whether the effect of the independent variable (X) (BIS) on the dependent variable (Y) (CUVINO categories: victim/aggressor) may be mediated by the mediating variables (M1; M2; M3), that is, the perceived emotional intelligence, with its three dimensions (attention, clarity, and emotional repair), including as covariates the sex and age variables. As shown in Figure 1, parameter (c') indicates the direct effect of X on Y, controlling for the mediating variable, (a) indicates the direct effect of X on M, (b) is the direct effect of M on Y, the indirect effect (ab) is the effect through the mediating variable, and the total effect (c) is the sum of the direct and indirect effects, when the mediator is excluded from the regression analysis.

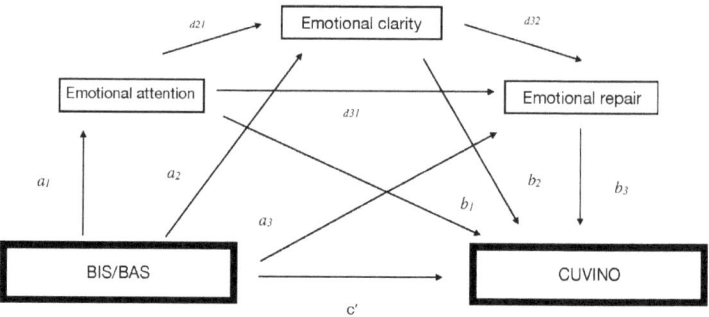

Figure 1. Conceptual and statistical scheme of the mediation of EI in the relationship between the BIS/BAS and the CUVINO factors for victimization and aggression.

3. Results

3.1. Descriptive Analyzes

Table 1 shows the count and percentage for each group according to the dimensions of the CUVINO questionnaire. A total of 83.1% of the sample reported some type of violence. Most of the violence reported was bidirectional (70.6%); that is, victim and aggressor were indistinctly reported by men and women. One-way violence was considerably lower (aggressor and non-victim: 3.7%; victim and non-aggressor: 12.5%). No victim or aggressor was reported in 13% of the total sample.

Table 1. Count and percentage for each group according to the dimensions of the CUVINO questionnaire.

	Victimization Profile			Aggression Profile	
	Non-Abuse	Technical Mistreatment	Mistreatment	Non-Perpetrator	Perpetrator
Overall	46 (16.9%)	153 (26.8%)	73 (56.3%)	70 (25.7%)	202 (74.3%)
Men	6	30	11	10	37
Women	40	123	62	60	165

Regarding the distribution by sex, there were no statistically significant differences for the victim profiles ($X^2 = 1.407$; $p = 0.495$), and no relationship was observed for aggression profiles either ($X^2 = 0.591$, $p = 0.442$).

Table 2 shows the descriptive statistics corresponding to age, emotional intelligence, and BIS/BAS for each group according to the type of intimate partner violence and total sample.

Table 2. Descriptive statistics corresponding to age, emotional intelligence, and the BIS/BAS for each group according to the type of couple violence and total sample.

	Victimization Profile						Aggression Profile				Overall	
	Non-Abuse		Technical Mistreatment		Mistreatment		Non-Perpetrator		Perpetrator			
	M	SD	M	SD	M	SD	M	SD	M	SD	M	SD
Age	20.70	2.45	20.63	2.28	21.84	2.83	20.31	1.92	21.19	2.66	20.97	2.51
Emotional attention	30.54	6.11	29.99	6.03	29.73	6.31	30.86	5.85	29.72	6.18	30.01	6.11
Emotional clarity	28.04	6.83	26.71	6.79	24.32	7.13	27.67	6.35	25.83	7.14	26.30	6.98
Emotional repair	28.15	6.60	25.50	6.95	24.98	6.55	26.83	6.52	25.46	6.95	25.81	6.85
BIS	35.76	6.05	35.03	5.81	34.22	5.35	35.11	6.10	34.88	5.61	34.94	5.73
BAS	39.48	3.17	38.32	4.09	37.60	4.10	39.70	3.89	37.85	3.92	38.32	3.99

In the victimization profile (abuse, technical abuse, and no abuse), significant differences regarding age were observed ($F = 6.182$; $p = 0.002$). Specifically, the maltreated were older than the non-maltreated ($p = 0.045$, $d = 1.1$) and the technically mistreated ($p = 0.002$, $d = 1.2$). Regarding behavioral sensitivity, significant differences were found between groups (abused, technical abuse, and no abuse) for the BAS variable ($F = 3.170$; $p = 0.044$), but no differences were observed in the BIS ($F = 1.069$; $p = 0.345$). Finally, regarding the EI dimensions, differences were observed between the victimization groups (mistreated, technical abuse, and non-abuse) in two dimensions: emotional clarity ($F = 4.746$; $p = 0.009$) and emotional repair ($F = 3.426$; $p = 0.034$). Pairwise comparisons showed differences between the abused and non-abused groups in the following dimensions: emotional clarity ($p = 0.014$; $d = 3.71$) and emotional repair ($p = 0.042$; $d = 3.1$), and between technical abuse and abused in the emotional clarity dimension ($p = 0.046$, $d = 2.3$). In all cases, the maltreated group obtained worse scores on the scales analyzed, followed by the technical maltreatment group, and the best results were observed in the non-abuse group. In summary, no differences between abused and non-abused were observed in the BIS. Abused people's scores were lower on the BAS scale, and they also obtained lower scores on the EI dimensions of clarity and repair. The scores of the technically mistreated group were lower than those of the mistreated group.

In the aggression profile, significant differences were observed regarding the factor age, with the aggressors being older than the non-aggressors (t = −2.965; p = 0.003). On the other hand, in terms of behavioral sensitivity, significant differences were observed between perpetrators and non-perpetrators on the BAS scale (t = 3.416; p = 0.001; d = 1.85), with non-aggressors showing higher scores. On the BIS scale, no significant differences were observed (t = 0.299; p = 0.765: d = 0.23). Finally, regarding the aggressors and non-aggressors EI, no significant differences were observed in the attention and emotional repair dimensions, although there was a trend of higher scores in the non-abused group compared with the abused group (t = 1.914; p = 0.057; d = 1.84).

The correlations between the three emotional intelligence dimensions (attention, clarity, and emotional repair), the BIS/BAS, age, and the two dimensions of the CUVINO (victimization and perpetration) were also analyzed (see Table 3).

Regarding the victimization profile, a negative correlation was observed between the BAS and the sexual- and coercive-type victims. The BIS negatively correlated with being a sexual victim, humiliation, and detachment. Regarding the EI dimensions, there was a negative correlation between the clarity dimension and each type of victim, while the emotional repair dimension was negatively correlated with being a sexual victim and a victim of detachment. Therefore, the lower the BIS score, the higher the victimization, and the higher the victimization, the lower the EI. That is, in the couple violence victims, the BIS and EI variables correlated negatively.

In the perpetration profile, the BAS was negatively correlated with being a sexual aggressor, humiliation, detachment, and coercive violence. However, the BIS was not correlated with the types of aggressors. Regarding the EI dimensions, a negative correlation was observed between attention and emotional clarity in detachment aggression. That is, the higher the detachment aggression, the lower the attention and emotional clarity. In the emotional repair dimension, no correlation was observed with any type of aggression.

3.2. Mediation Analysis

After the preliminary and correlation analyses, we aimed to study the mediation process of EI in the relationship between the BIS/BAS and the role of the victim or aggressor. In the mediation analysis, the mediator variable (EI) should correlate both with the dependent variable (victimization/perpetration) and the independent variable (BAS/BAS).

According to our analyses, EI was not correlated with the BAS, so this variable was not included in the mediation analyses. However, EI was significantly correlated with the BIS and victimization, but the BIS was not correlated with perpetration. Therefore, the mediation analysis was conducted to explore if the EI mediates the effects of the BIS on the related types of victims, that is, sexual, humiliation, and detachment.

Table 3. Correlation between emotional intelligence, BIS/BAS, and CUVINO factors for victimization and aggression.

		1	2	3	4	5	6	7	8	9	10	11	12	13	14
	1. Emotional attention	-													
	2. Emotional clarity	0.443 **	-												
	3. Emotional repair	0.200 **	0.436 **	-											
	4. BIS	−0.134 *	0.277 **	0.371 **	-										
	5. BAS	−0.073	0.045	0.044	0.031	-									
Victim	6. Physical	−0.049	−0.125 *	0.008	−0.024	−0.09	-								
	7. Sexual	0.002	−0.142 *	−0.140 *	−0.175 **	−0.128 *	0.492 **	-							
	8. Humiliation	−0.003	−0.147 *	−0.094	−0.142 *	−0.044	0.400 **	0.365 **	-						
	9. Detachment	−0.019	−0.247 **	−0.192 **	−0.186 **	−0.11	0.232 **	0.303 **	0.447 **	-					
	10. Coercion	−0.013	−0.139 *	−0.049	−0.082	−0.202 **	0.378 **	0.386 **	0.421 **	0.283 **	-				
Aggressor	11. Physical	−0.001	0.016	0.018	0.095	−0.09	0.440 **	0.255 **	0.198 **	0.173 **	0.168 **	-			
	12. Sexual	−0.021	−0.039	−0.012	0.037	−0.137 *	0.229 **	0.353 **	0.153 *	0.049	0.174 **	0.251 **	-		
	13. Humiliation	−0.013	−0.086	−0.076	0.005	−0.197 **	0.056	0.067	0.519 **	0.282 **	0.168 **	0.201 **	0.178 **	-	
	14. Detachment	−0.148 *	−0.214 **	−0.021	−0.041	−0.154 *	0.066	0.151 *	0.252 **	0.443 **	0.252 **	0.114	0.127 *	0.242 **	-
	15. Coercion	0.091	0.006	−0.117	−0.07	−0.197 **	0.104	0.136 *	0.233 **	0.233 **	0.500 **	0.312 **	0.098	0.274 **	0.185 **

* $p < 0.05$; ** $p < 0.00$.

Thus, three serial mediation models were analyzed to determine if the BIS scores and EI dimensions are related to sexual victimization (model 1), humiliation victimization (model 2), and detachment (model 3). Age and sex were considered covariates (Table 4).

Table 4. Results of the analysis of mediation of emotional intelligence in the relationship between BIS and sexual victimization (model 1), humiliation (model 2), and detachment (model 3), including as covariates age and sex.

Path	Coefficient	HE	BootLLCI	BootULCI	t	p
Model 1 (Sexual Victimization)						
Total effect (c)	−0.0339	0.0109	−0.0554	−0.0124	−30.995	0.0021
Direct effect (c')	−0.0242	0.0122	−0.0482	−0.0001	−1.9791	0.0488
a_1	−0.1036	0.0663	−0.234	0.0269	−15.631	0.1192
a_2	0.3978	0.0644	0.2710	0.5246	6.177	0.000
a_3	0.3324	0.0695	0.1956	0.4692	4.784	0.000
b_1	0.0077	0.0118	−0.0155	0.0309	0.6537	0.513
b_2	−0.0155	0.0108	−368	0.0059	−1.426	0.154
b_3	−0.0088	0.0103	−0.0291	0.0116	−0.8509	0.3956
d_{21}	0.5694	0.0591	0.4531	0.6858	9.636	0.000
d_{31}	0.1417	0.0692	0.0054	0.2781	20.469	0.0417
d_{32}	0.2923	0.0618	0.1707	0.4139	4.732	0.000
Indirect effects	Effects	HE	BootLLCI	BootULCI		
Total indirect effect	−0.0242	0.0050	−0.0199	−0.0002		
Model 2 (Humiliation Victimization)						
Path	Coefficient	HE	BootLLCI	BootULCI	t	p
Total effect (c)	−0.0281	0.0112	−0.0501	−0.0061	−2.5128	0.0126
Direct effect (c')	−0.0193	0.0125	−0.0439	0.0053	−1.5439	0.1238
a_1	−0.1036	0.0663	−0.234	0.0269	−1.5631	0.1192
a_2	0.3978	0.0644	0.271	0.5246	6.1776	0.000
a_3	0.3324	0.0695	0.1956	0.4692	4.7841	0.000
b_1	0.0094	0.012	−0.0143	0.0331	0.778	0.4373
b_2	−0.0208	0.0111	−0.0427	0.001	−1.8776	0.0615
b_3	−0.0019	0.0106	−0.0227	0.0189	−0.1797	0.8576
d_{21}	0.5694	0.0591	0.4531	0.6858	9.6368	0.000
d_{31}	0.1417	0.0692	0.0054	0.2781	2.0469	0.0417
d_{32}	0.2923	0.0618	0.1707	0.4139	4.7323	0.000
Indirect effects	Effects	HE	BootLLCI	BootULCI		
Total indirect effect	−0.0088	0.0055	−0.0198	0.0018		
Model 3 (Detachment Victimization)						
Path	Coefficient	HE	BootLLCI	BootULCI	t	p
Total effect (c)	−0.0473	0.0153	−0.0774	−0.0172	−3.0937	0.0022
Direct effect (c')	−0.0226	0.0167	−1.3524	0.1774	−0.0556	0.0103
a_1	−0.1036	0.0663	−0.2340	0.0269	−1.563	0.1192
a_2	0.3978	0.0644	0.271	0.5246	6.1776	0.000
a_3	0.3324	0.0695	0.1956	0.4692	4.7841	0.000
b_1	0.0203	0.0161	−0.0114	0.0521	1.2601	0.2087
b_2	−0.0465	0.0149	−0.0758	−0.0172	−3.124	0.002
b_3	−0.0163	0.0142	−0.0442	0.0116	−1.1515	0.2506
d_{21}	0.5694	0.0591	0.4531	0.6858	9.636	0.000
d_{31}	0.1417	0.0692	0.0054	0.2781	2.0469	0.0417
d_{32}	0.2923	0.0618	0.1707	0.4139	4.7323	0.000
Indirect effects	Effects	HE	BootLLCI	BootULCI		
Total indirect effect	−0.0247	0.0084	−0.0419	−0.0088		
Ind2: $a_2 b_2$	−0.0185	0.0068	−0.033	−0.0064		

Notes: Abbreviations: BootLLCI: bootstrapping lower limit confidence interval; BootULCI: bootstrapping upper limit confidence interval; HE: standard error. Model: 6. Y: sexual victimization/humiliation victimization/detachment victimization. X: BIS. M1: emotional attention. M2: emotional clarity. M3: emotional repair. Covariates: age and sex. N = 272.

We detail here the results of the different linear regression analyses considering the EI dimensions and the independent variable (BIS). Regarding emotional attention, the percentage of variance explained by the BIS (a_1) and the covariates was 4.06%, although only the factor sex was significant ($B = 2.414$; $t = 2.438$; $p = 0.0154$). Regarding emotional clarity, the percentage of variance explained by the BIS and the covariates was 31.54%. In this case, significant differences were observed in the BIS (a_2) and emotional attention (d_{21}), with the factors sex and age showing no significance ($p > 0.05$). Concerning emotional repair, the percentage of variance explained by the BIS was 27.90%, with the covariate sex being significant ($B = -2.147$; $t = -2.192$; $p = 0.029$), as well as the variables BIS (a_3), attention emotional (d_{31}), and emotional clarity (d_{32}) (Table 3).

Regarding the results of the multiple linear regression analyses, considering EI and the BIS as predictor variables, the three types of victims with significant correlations were included.

First, for model 1 (sexual victimization), the BIS ($B = -0.0242$; $t = -1.979$; $p = 0.0488$) and the covariate age ($B = 0.0558$; $t = 2.283$; $p = 0.0232$) were significant factors, and they explained 6.26% of the total variance. In this model, the total effect of the BIS was significant. In addition, in this model, direct, but not indirect, effects of the BIS were observed.

Second, for model 2 (victimization by humiliation), the total variance explained was 3.98%, although here there were no significant differences, and we only found a trend of significance in emotional clarity (b_2) ($F = 0.0936$; $p = 0.093$). In this model, the total effect of the BIS was significant, while neither direct nor indirect effects were observed (Table 3).

Finally, for model 3 (detachment victimization), a significant effect was observed in the multiple linear regression analysis ($F = 4.434$; $p = 0.0003$). Emotional clarity (b_2) resulted in a significant variable explaining 9.12% of the total variance of the model in this type of victim (Table 3). In this model, the total effect of the BIS was significant, but no direct effects were observed. Lastly, in this model, we observed indirect effects of the BIS (X) on detachment victimization (Y), and these effects were mediated by emotional clarity (Figure 2 and Table 3). Therefore, the emotional clarity dimension in the victims due to detachment can be considered a mediator of the BIS. Thus, low levels of BIS are associated with poor emotional clarity and more indicators of victimization due to detachment.

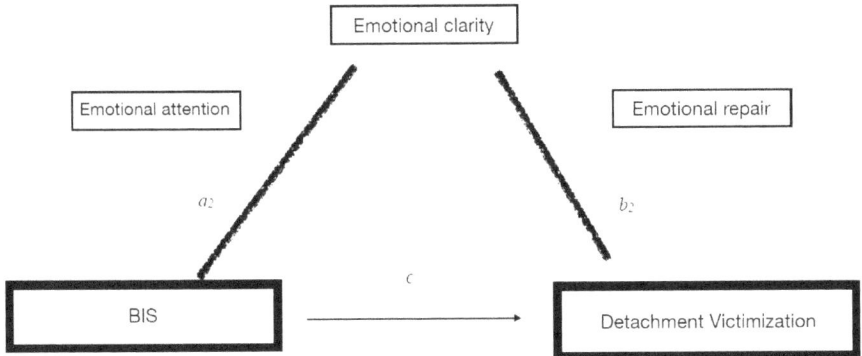

Figure 2. Mediation of EI in the relationship between the BIS/BAS and the CUVINO factors for victimization and aggression. Indirect effects corresponding to Model 3: BIS on detachment victimization.

4. Discussion

According to the descriptive analyses, the majority of reported abuse cases appear to be bidirectional, a trend consistent with previous studies [5–8,10,11,14–19]. This reciprocal pattern of violence is associated with the absence of discernible differences between men and women, both in terms of victim and aggressor profiles. In other words, both men and women can interchangeably be victims or aggressors in intimate partner violence.

Regarding the victimization profiles, distinctions emerged among different types of victims concerning behavioral sensitivity. Victims exhibited lower scores on the BAS scale, indicating a reduced sensitivity to incentives and goal-directed behavior. Consequently, victims reported lower levels of happiness and positive moods [32]. This is also true concerning the aggression profile, but in the opposite direction; that is, higher scores were found in the BAS scores of people who do not mistreat their partners. These people are sensitive to rewards, feel hope and euphoria, aim at accomplishing goals and finding happiness in their achievements, and, therefore, show more affection, feelings, and positive emotions [32].

In terms of EI, victims who reported abuse and technical mistreatment exhibited lower emotional clarity and emotional repair abilities. This implies a deficiency in understanding their own emotions and the emotions of others, which may hinder their ability to regulate emotions effectively (self-regulation). Consequently, victims with low EI experience personal discomfort. It is evident that victims tend to possess lower EI, aligning with the conclusions of Moreno et al. [37], who emphasize the importance of EI skills in preventing violence in young couples. In contrast, individuals who do not engage in aggression, particularly those who refrain from physical violence against their partners, displayed higher emotional clarity. This means they have a better grasp of their own emotions and the emotions of others, consistent with the results of Zapata [36], who demonstrated significantly lower EI levels in individuals perpetrating violence against their partners.

Regarding the correlations in the victimization profile, a negative correlation was observed between the BAS scores for sexual and coercive victims. High levels of sexual and coercive victimization correlated with low BAS activation. This is consistent with the results of Meyer et al. [31] since they reported that the BAS is also affected by situations of interpersonal threat because these involve the loss of rewards and incentives (in this case, the couple's relationship). Furthermore, sexual victimization, humiliation, and detachment correlated negatively with the BI, indicating that these types of victims do not perceive violence with their partners as a threat and do not pay attention to danger signals, even in high-threat situations [49]. It is worth noting that there is no established causal relationship between low BIS activation and high victimization. Low BIS levels may be linked to EI since all victim types exhibited a negative correlation with emotional clarity, implying a reduced ability to understand their own emotions and those of others. This lack of emotional clarity might explain why victims do not perceive intimate partner violence situations as threatening and do not process danger signals effectively. Concerning emotional repair, which involves self-regulation and the management of personal emotions, the same trend is observed. Victims of sexual victimization exhibited a negative correlation between detachment and the BIS. It is possible that low BIS levels in sexual victims are related to low EI levels because threatening situations may not be processed as such.

On the other hand, within the aggression profile and terms of behavioral sensitivity, sexual, humiliation, detachment, and coercive aggressors show lower scores in the BAS, which means that they do not effectively process information related to incentives and rewards, and as a result, they do not generate positive feelings such as hope and euphoria. In this aggression profile, we also found higher BIS scores; that is, these aggressors process the information as highly threatening and triggering anxiety and excitement, and they focus attention on danger signals [32]. The EI of the aggressors due to detachment negatively correlated with attention and emotional clarity. We found that low EI is associated with aggression, which means that the aggressors, at least due to detachment, have a poor ability to understand their own emotions and the emotions of others, and this low emotional clarity may be related to the use of violence as a way of resolving conflicts in the couple, in the absence of healthy strategies.

Finally, in the context of mediation analysis, our results demonstrate that in victims of detachment violence, EI, particularly the emotional clarity dimension, acts as a mediator of the BIS. Previous studies have shown that BIS activity moderates the relationship between threat and anxiety [49]. Meyer et al. [31] highlighted the effect of BIS sensitivity in threatened relationships, noting that low partner threat levels are not associated with distress, even with high BIS levels, whereas high threat levels and high BIS levels are closely linked to distress. High BIS sensitivity has previously been associated with distress in various stressful situations [49–53]. The perception of situations as stressful or highly threatening appears to be essential for triggering anxiety.

Our results suggest that threat perception might in turn be influenced by EI, specifically by emotional clarity. Victims of couple violence due to detachment exhibited low emotional clarity, implying a diminished ability to understand personal emotions and the emotions of others. This may prevent victims from interpreting violence as a threat to the relationship or as a stressful situation in general. Consequently, the BIS response is not triggered, as the situation is not perceived as dangerous to personal well-being [31].

This study had certain limitations. Expanding the sample to include specific sex and age groups and collecting data from nationally representative samples would be beneficial. Longitudinal studies would also be valuable, as cross-sectional studies may limit the generalizability of the findings. Additionally, it is important to acknowledge that self-reports and observational studies can introduce biases.

Nevertheless, this study significantly contributes to understanding the motivational and emotional processes involved in dating violence, shedding light on potential psychological interventions.

5. Conclusions

The findings of this study reveal that there are no significant differences in young couple violence between sex, as both men and women can be victims and aggressors interchangeably, demonstrating a bidirectional pattern of violence. However, differences are observed concerning age, as both victimization and perpetration rates increase with age.

Regarding behavioral sensitivity, both victims and aggressors show low BAS sensitivity, while individuals who do not engage in abuse behavior towards their partners display high BAS sensitivity.

In terms of EI, it has been observed that victims of abuse and technical abuse, as well as perpetrators, tend to have lower EI levels compared to individuals who do not commit violence against their partners, who show higher levels of EI.

Additionally, sexual and coercive victimization are associated with reduced BAS activation, whereas sexual, humiliation, and detachment victimization are linked to lower BIS activation. Furthermore, all types of victimization are correlated with less emotional clarity. In the case of aggressors, including those involved in sexual, humiliation, detachment, and coercion, lower BAS activation and higher BIS activation are observed. Detachment aggression is specifically associated with poor emotional clarity.

Finally, the mediation analyses have revealed that emotional clarity, an EI dimension, acts as a mediator of BIS activation in victims of detachment. Based on these results, the implementation of programs for the acquisition of EI skills in young people of both sexes might be a useful approach for this kind of victim. Specifically, we consider it important that nursery school programs train students in EI, as this is fundamental to being able to identify and understand their own emotions as well as those of the people around them. In addition, psychotherapists need to consider the important tool that EI represents in the fight against intimate partner violence, both for men and women.

Author Contributions: Conceptualization, M.P.S.-A., A.M.-C. and J.R.A.-B.; methodology, M.P.S.-A., A.M.-C. and J.R.A.-B.; formal analysis, M.P.S.-A., A.M.-C. and J.R.A.-B.; writing—original draft preparation, review, and editing, M.P.S.-A., A.M.-C. and J.R.A.-B. All authors have read and agreed to the published version of the manuscript.

Funding: This research received no external funding.

Institutional Review Board Statement: The study was conducted according to the guidelines of the Declaration of Helsinki, and ethical review and approval were waived for this study, because they were not applicable.

Informed Consent Statement: Informed consent was obtained from all subjects involved in the study.

Data Availability Statement: The dataset is available in the repository.

Conflicts of Interest: The authors declare no conflict of interest.

References

1. McLaughlin, J.; O'Carroll, R.E.; O'Connor, R.C. Intimate Partner Abuse and Suicidality: A Systematic Review. *Clin. Psychol. Rev.* **2012**, *32*, 677–689. [CrossRef] [PubMed]
2. Loinaz, I.; Ortiz-Tallo, M.; Sánchez, L.M.; Ferragut, M. Clasificación Multiaxial de Agresores de Pareja En Centros Penitenciarios. *Int. J. Clin. Health Psychol.* **2011**, *11*, 249–268.
3. Rodriguez Biezma, M.J.R. Violencia Hacia La Pareja: Revisión Teórica. *Psicopatol. Clínica Leg. Forense* **2007**, *7*, 77–95.
4. Paíno-Quesada, S.; Aguilera-Jiménez, N.; Rodríguez-Franco, L.; Rodríguez-Díaz, F.; Alameda-Bailén, J. Conflicto Adolescente y Relaciones de Pareja de Adultos Jóvenes: Direccionalidad de La Violencia. *Rev. Int. Investig. Psicol.* **2020**, *13*, 36–48.
5. Zamora-Damián, G.; Alvídrez Villegas, S.; Aizpitarte, A.; Rojas-Solís, J.L. Prevalencia de Violencia En El Noviazgo En Una Muestra de Varones Adolescentes Mexicanos. *Rev. Psicol. Cienc. Comport. Unidad Académica Cienc. Jurídicas Soc.* **2018**, *9*, 30–53. [CrossRef]
6. Alegría del Angel, M.; Rodríguez Barraza, A. Violencia Mutua En El Noviazgo: Perfil Psicosocial Víctima-Victimario En Universitarios. *Psicol. Salud* **2017**, *27*, 231–244.
7. Archer, J. Sex Differences in Aggression between Heterosexual Partners: A Meta-Analytic Review. *Psychol. Bull.* **2000**, *126*, 651. [CrossRef]
8. Arnoso, A.; Ibabe, I.; Arnoso, M.; Elgorriaga, E. El sexismo como predictor de la violencia de pareja en un contexto multicultural. *Anu. Psicol. Jurídica* **2017**, *27*, 9–20. [CrossRef]
9. Chen, M.; Chan, K.L. Characteristics of Intimate Partner Violence in China: Gender Symmetry, Mutuality, and Associated Factors. *J. Interpers. Violence* **2021**, *36*, NP6867–NP6889. [CrossRef]
10. Graña Gómez, J.L.; Cuenca Montesino, M.L. Prevalence of Psychological and Physical Intimate Partner Aggression in Madrid (Spain): A Dyadic Analysis. *Psicothema* **2014**, *26*, 343–348.
11. Rojas-Solís, J.L.; Morales, L.A.; Juarros Basterretxea, J.; Herrero Olaizola, J.; Rodríguez Díaz, F.J. Propiedades psicométricas del Inventario de Estilos de Resolución de Conflictos en jóvenes mexicanos. *Rev. Iberoam. Psicol. Salud* **2019**, *10*, 15–26.
12. Straus, M.A. Dominance and Symmetry in Partner Violence by Male and Female University Students in 32 Nations. *Child. Youth Serv. Rev.* **2008**, *30*, 252–275. [CrossRef]
13. Conroy, E.; Willmott, D.; Murphy, A.; Widanaralalage, B.K. Does Perpetrator Gender Influence Attitudes towards Intimate Partner Violence (IPV)? Examining the Relationship between Male-Perpetrated and Female-Perpetrated IPV Attitudes among a Sample of UK Young Adults. *Ment. Health Soc. Incl.* **2023**. [CrossRef]
14. Johnson, W.L.; Giordano, P.C.; Manning, W.D.; Longmore, M.A. The Age-IPV Curve: Changes in Intimate Partner Violence Perpetration during Adolescence and Young Adulthood. *J. Youth Adolesc.* **2015**, *44*, 708–726. [CrossRef] [PubMed]
15. Melander, L.A.; Noel, H.; Tyler, K.A. Bidirectional, Unidirectional, and Nonviolence: A Comparison of the Predictors among Partnered Young Adults. *Violence Vict.* **2010**, *25*, 617–630. [CrossRef]
16. Rodríguez Pérez, S. Violencia En Parejas Jóvenes: Estudio Preliminar Sobre Su Prevalencia Y Motivos1/Dating Violence: Preliminary Study of Prevalence and Justification/Violência Entre Casais Jovens: Estudo Preliminar Sobre Sua Prevalência E Motivos. *Pedagog. Soc.* **2015**, 251–275. [CrossRef]
17. Rubio-Garay, F.; López-González, M.Á.; Saúl, L.Á.; Sánchez-Elvira-Paniagua, Á. Direccionalidad Y Expresión De La Violencia En Las Relaciones De Noviazgo De Los Jóvenes/Directionality and Violence Expression Indating Relationship of Young People. *Acción Psicol.* **2012**, *9*, 61–70. [CrossRef]
18. Rubio-Garay, F.; Carrasco Ortiz, M.Á.; García-Rodríguez, B. Moral Disengagement and Violence in Adolescent and Young Dating Relationships: An Exploratory Study. *Rev. Argent. Clín. Psicol.* **2019**, *28*, 22–31.
19. Straus, M.A. Why the Overwhelming Evidence on Partner Physical Violence by Women Has Not Been Perceived and Is Often Denied. *J. Aggress. Maltreat. Trauma* **2009**, *18*, 552–571. [CrossRef]
20. Johnson, M.P. Gender and Types of Intimate Partner Violence: A Response to an Anti-Feminist Literature Review. *Aggress. Violent Behav.* **2011**, *16*, 289–296. [CrossRef]
21. Muñoz Rivas, M.J.; Graña Gómez, J.L.; O'Leary, D.K.; González Lozano, P. Physical and Psychological Aggression in Dating Relationships in Spanish University Students. "Agresión Física y Psicológica En Las Relaciones de Noviazgo En Universitarios Españoles". *Psicothema* **2007**, *19*, 102–107. [PubMed]
22. Rubio-Garay, F.; López González, M.Á.; Carrasco Ortiz, M.Á.; Amor Andrés, P.J. Prevalencia de la violencia en el noviazgo: Una revisión sistemática. *Papeles Psicól.* **2017**, *38*, 135–147.
23. Echeburúa, E. Crítica de Artículos: Sobre el Papel del Género en la Violencia de Pareja contra la Mujer. Comentario a Ferrer-Pérez y Bosch-Fiol, 2019. *Anu. Psicol. Jurídica* **2019**, *29*, 77–79. [CrossRef]
24. Ibabe, I.; Arnoso, A.; Elgorriaga, E. Child-to-Parent Violence as an Intervening Variable in the Relationship between Inter-Parental Violence Exposure and Dating Violence. *Int. J. Environ. Res. Public Health* **2020**, *17*, 1514. [CrossRef] [PubMed]

25. Cuadrado-Gordillo, I.; Fernández-Antelo, I.; Parra, G.M.-M. Search for the Profile of the Victim of Adolescent Dating Violence: An Intersection of Cognitive, Emotional, and Behavioral Variables. *Int. J. Environ. Res. Public Health* **2020**, *17*, 8004. [CrossRef] [PubMed]
26. Gray, J.A. The Psychophysiological Basis of Introversion-Extraversion. *Behav. Res. Ther.* **1970**, *8*, 249–266. [CrossRef] [PubMed]
27. Gray, J.A. *The Psychology of Fear and Stress*; Cambridge University Press: Cambridge, UK, 1987.
28. Gray, J.A. A Critique of Eysenck's Theory of Personality. In *A Model for Personality*; Eysenck, H.J., Ed.; Springer: New York, NY, USA, 1981; pp. 246–276, ISBN 978-3-642-67785-4.
29. Corr, P.J. Reinforcement Sensitivity Theory (RST): Introduction. In *The Reinforcement Sensitivity Theory of Personality*; Cambridge University Press: New York, NY, USA, 2008; pp. 1–43, ISBN 978-0-521-61736-9.
30. Carver, C.S.; Meyer, B.; Antoni, M.H. Responsiveness to Threats and Incentives, Expectancy of Recurrence, and Distress and Disengagement: Moderator Effects in Women with Early Stage Breast Cancer. *J. Consult. Clin. Psychol.* **2000**, *68*, 965. [CrossRef] [PubMed]
31. Meyer, B.; Olivier, L.; Roth, D.A. Please Don't Leave Me! BIS/BAS, Attachment Styles, and Responses to a Relationship Threat. *Personal. Individ. Differ.* **2005**, *38*, 151–162. [CrossRef]
32. Merchán-Clavellino, A.; Alameda-Bailén, J.R.; Zayas García, A.; Guil, R. Mediating Effect of Trait Emotional Intelligence Between the Behavioral Activation System (BAS)/Behavioral Inhibition System (BIS) and Positive and Negative Affect. *Front. Psychol.* **2019**, *10*, 424. [CrossRef]
33. Extremera Pacheco, N.; Fernández Berrocal, P. Inteligencia Emocional Percibida y Diferencias Individuales En El Meta-Conocimiento de Los Estados Emocionales: Una Revisión de Los Estudios Con El TMMS. *Ansiedad Estrés* **2005**, *11*, 101–122.
34. Mayer, J.D.; Salovey, P. What Is Emotional Intelligence? In *Emotional Development and Emotional Intelligence: Educational Implications*, 2nd ed.; Basic: New York, NY, USA, 1997; pp. 3–31.
35. García González, B.; Quezada Berumen, L. del C. Inteligencia Emocional Como Predictora de La Satisfacción En La Relación Entre Jóvenes Víctimas y No Víctimas de Violencia En El Noviazgo. *Summa Psicol. UST* **2020**, *17*, 4.
36. Zapata Santamaria, C.W. *Inteligencia Emocional y Violencia en la Pareja en Jovenes Pertenecientes a la Policia de Chiclayo*; Universidad Señor de Sipán: Chiclayo, Peru, 2019.
37. Moreno, J.M.; Blazquez Alonso, M.; Garcia-Baamonde Sanchez, M.E.; Guerrero Barona, E. Psychological Abuse in Young Couples: Risk Factors. *J. Soc. Serv. Res.* **2011**, *37*, 555–570.
38. Bacon, A.M.; Corr, P.J. Motivating Emotional Intelligence: A Reinforcement Sensitivity Theory (RST) Perspective. *Motiv. Emot.* **2017**, *41*, 254–264. [CrossRef]
39. Li, Y.; Xu, Y.; Chen, Z. Effects of the Behavioral Inhibition System (BIS), Behavioral Activation System (BAS), and Emotion Regulation on Depression: A One-Year Follow-up Study in Chinese Adolescents. *Psychiatry Res.* **2015**, *230*, 287–293. [CrossRef]
40. Rodríguez-Díaz, F.J.; Herrero, J.; Rodríguez-Franco, L.; Bringas-Molleda, C.; Paíno-Quesada, S.G.; Pérez, B. Validation of Dating Violence Questionnarie-R (DVQ-R). *Int. J. Clin. Health Psychol.* **2017**, *17*, 77–84. [CrossRef] [PubMed]
41. López-Cepero, J.; Fabelo, H.E.; Rodríguez-Franco, L.; Rodríguez-Díaz, F.J. The Dating Violence Questionnaire: Validation of the Cuestionario de Violencia de Novios Using a College Sample from the United States. *Violence Vict.* **2016**, *31*, 438–456. [CrossRef] [PubMed]
42. Presaghi, F.; Manca, M.; Rodriguez-Franco, L.; Curcio, G. A Questionnaire for the Assessment of Violent Behaviors in Young Couples: The Italian Version of Dating Violence Questionnaire (DVQ). *PLoS ONE* **2015**, *10*, e0126089. [CrossRef] [PubMed]
43. Torrubia, R.; Ávila, C.; Moltó, J.; Caseras, X. The Sensitivity to Punishment and Sensitivity to Reward Questionnaire (SPSRQ) as a Measure of Gray's Anxiety and Impulsivity Dimensions. *Personal. Individ. Differ.* **2001**, *31*, 837–862. [CrossRef]
44. Caseras, X.; Àvila, C.; Torrubia, R. The Measurement of Individual Differences in Behavioural Inhibition and Behavioural Activation Systems: A Comparison of Personality Scales. *Personal. Individ. Differ.* **2003**, *34*, 999–1013. [CrossRef]
45. Salovey, P.; Mayer, J.D.; Goldman, S.L.; Turvey, C.; Palfai, T.P. Emotional Attention, Clarity, and Repair: Exploring Emotional Intelligence Using the Trait Meta-Mood Scale. In *Emotion, Disclosure, and Health*; American Psychological Association: Washington, DC, USA, 1995; pp. 125–154.
46. Fernández-Berrocal, P.; Extremera, N.; Ramos, N. Validity and Reliability of the Spanish Modified Version of the Trait Meta-Mood Scale. *Psychol. Rep.* **2004**, *94*, 751–755. [CrossRef]
47. Cohen, J. *Statistical Power Analysis for the Behavioral Sciences*; Routledge: Oxfordshire, UK, 2013; ISBN 978-0-203-77158-7.
48. Hayes, A.F. *Model Templates for PROCESS for SPSS and SAS*; Guilford Press: New York, NY, USA, 2013.
49. Carver, C.S.; White, T.L. Behavioral Inhibition, Behavioral Activation, and Affective Responses to Impending Reward and Punishment: The BIS/BAS Scales. *J. Personal. Soc. Psychol.* **1994**, *67*, 319. [CrossRef]
50. Johnson, S.L.; Turner, R.J.; Iwata, N. BIS/BAS Levels and Psychiatric Disorder: An Epidemiological Study. *J. Psychopathol. Behav. Assess.* **2003**, *25*, 25–36. [CrossRef]
51. Carver, C.S.; Sutton, S.K.; Scheier, M.F. Action, Emotion, and Personality: Emerging Conceptual Integration. *Personal. Soc. Psychol. Bull.* **2000**, *26*, 741–751. [CrossRef]

52. Heponiemi, T.; Keltikangas-Järvinen, L.; Puttonen, S.; Ravaja, N. BIS/BAS Sensitivity and Self-Rated Affects during Experimentally Induced Stress. *Personal. Individ. Differ.* **2003**, *34*, 943–957. [CrossRef]
53. Kasch, K.L.; Rottenberg, J.; Arnow, B.A.; Gotlib, I.H. Behavioral Activation and Inhibition Systems and the Severity and Course of Depression. *J. Abnorm. Psychol.* **2002**, *111*, 589. [CrossRef]

Disclaimer/Publisher's Note: The statements, opinions and data contained in all publications are solely those of the individual author(s) and contributor(s) and not of MDPI and/or the editor(s). MDPI and/or the editor(s) disclaim responsibility for any injury to people or property resulting from any ideas, methods, instructions or products referred to in the content.

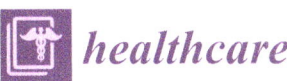 healthcare

Article

Prevalence and Characteristics of Sexual Victimization among Gay and Bisexual Men: A Preliminary Study in Spain

Xavier Calvet * and Leonor M. Cantera

Social Psychology Area, Department of Social Psychology, Universitat Autònoma de Barcelona (UAB), 08193 Bellaterra, Barcelona, Spain; leonor.cantera@uab.cat
* Correspondence: francescxavier.calveti@autonoma.cat or xavier.calvet.colome@gmail.com

Abstract: Sexual violence is an understudied issue in the population of gay and bisexual men, although the existing articles to date demonstrate that it is a problem that merits public attention. This study aims to approach the problem of invisibility around the matter, as well as presenting a number of variables that have been usually overlooked in Spanish research or have not been assessed at all. Lifetime sexual victimization, sociodemographic characteristics, situational characteristics and social support were examined among 550 gay and bisexual males living in Spain using a self-administrated questionnaire. Results analysis show that 90.00% (87.18–92.38%) of participants reported at least one experience of unwanted insinuation, 87.27% (84.19–89.94%) reported at least one experience of sexual coercion, 64.00% (59.83–68.02%) reported at least one experience of sexual assault, and specifically 19.82% (16.57–23.40%) reported being raped during their lifetime. Significant differences have been found between some categories regarding gender identity, sexual orientation, age, race/ethnicity and educational level. Overall, these results showcase sexual violence as a pervasive problem in the Spanish gay and bisexual community.

Keywords: sexual violence; intimate partner violence; gay; bisexual; transsexual; victimization; Spain

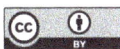

1. Introduction

Sexual violence (SV) is defined by the World Health Organization (WHO) as any unwanted sexual act directed against a person, regardless of the aggressor's relationship with the victim and the context in which it occurs [1]. The forms of SV may include sexual assault, unwanted sexual advances, sexual coercion or sexual abuse. Thus, the term encompasses a wide variety of circumstances and configurations. For example, it includes rape within marriage and by strangers, as well as abuse of minors and of persons who are mentally or physically incapacitated. Unwanted sexual advances or sexual harassment, refusal to use protection against pregnancy or sexually transmitted diseases (STDs), as well as many others, are also included in their definition of SV. The main reasons for the study of SV are the physical and/or psychological consequences suffered by the victims. Other than the possible injuries produced by any violent experience, unwanted pregnancy and the transmission of STDs, the appearance of phobias, depressive and anxious symptomatology, impoverished self-esteem, sexual dysfunctions, social difficulties and post-traumatic stress disorder are the most prominent consequences for victims of SV [2]. For all these reasons, SV is considered a social emergency that can have serious health consequences.

Historically, SV has been conceptualized as a type of violence carried out by a man against a woman, based on a conception of power that, to a large extent, characterized the second feminist wave. This perspective argues that men use violence against women as an extension of the patriarchal structure and as an expression of control and power over them [3], focusing on the intersection of class and gender systems of oppression [4]. This theory received several criticisms. One of the most notable was from black feminism, which added the intersection of the racial/ethnic axis to take into account the particularities experienced by black women in the patriarchal and capitalist system since the traditional conception neglected such experiences [5]. Gradually, axes of oppression were added, whose intersection explained the particular experiences in terms of race/ethnicity, class, gender, age, sexuality, functional diversity, religion, etc. Specifically, intersectionality, as a branch of feminist theory, is concerned with identifying how various systems of power, operating at multiple levels (e.g., structural and interpersonal), combine and interact to confer disproportionate risk on populations with marginalized social identities [6]. Although stated in a very brief and simplified way, as it is not the main focus of this paper, we can see how the interest in the intersectional study of SV, as opposed to the traditional feminist theory, allows us to explain why some men might suffer victimization experiences. Even so, only a small part of the existing research on intimate partner violence and SV to date is grounded in the theoretical framework and methods of intersectionality [7], so the collective of gay and bisexual men (GBM), the subject of this study, has been particularly neglected. In relation to this, most studies based on the feminist framework have neglected men rape, and this maintains and reinforces patriarchal power relations and hegemonic masculinities [8]. In terms of sexual orientation, we could conclude that the study of SV still has a strong heterosexist bias [9].

Additional resistances can be identified that block the study of SV in this group. First, there exist a number of male rape myths and beliefs, which are organized into three main themes: denial myths ("men cannot be raped"), blaming myths ("men are responsible for being raped") and trauma myths ("men who are raped do not really suffer discomfort") [10]. The internalization of these beliefs would result in a decrease in interest in the subject by the scientific community and, consequently, a reduction in the number of studies addressing it. Second, the reluctance on the part of researchers to address unwanted or non-consensual sex in GBM, as well as in any other LGTBIQA+ group, could be related to an attempt to avoid reproducing heterosexist ideas that define sexual minorities as deviant, criminal, predatory, pedophilic, and rapist [11]. In fact, there is an intention on the part of the scientific community to reconceptualize same-gender sexual relationships as healthy, legitimate and non-essentially violent in order to debunk such myths [12], which although necessary, inevitably obscures the violence that might occur within the collective. Third, given the HIV epidemic, there was a great interest and need to focus the study of men who have sex with men on the prevention of HIV transmission. Although this branch of study is interested in exploring SV [13], it tends to prioritize addressing the effects of HIV; an incomplete part of the comprehensive study of SV in the collective. In fact, there is an overwhelming frequency in which certain variables appear in the quantitative literature related to the GBM collective, especially putting the focus on HIV and STDs [14]. The study of these variables is indispensable, but it is also necessary to expand the study of health and well-being among the GBM population to understand many other factors that can be crucial, such as SV.

Although interest in the quantitative and qualitative study of sexual violence in GBM has increased in recent decades, it has been mostly in the context of intragender violence or domestic violence in same-sex relationships [15,16], in addition to prison-associated SV [17] and child abuse [18]. In fact, to our knowledge, there is no Spanish study at present that addresses sexual violence in the GBM collective, although there are a few that do discuss intragender violence [19,20].

There are, however, more international studies on sexual violence focused on the GBM population, regardless of the bond between victim and perpetrator. Some of their results report a 35.2% prevalence of non-consensual sex among men who have sex with men [21], 54.0% prevalence of sexual assault [22], 15.5% of physical SV, sexual assault, and stalking in the past 6 months [23], frequencies for sexual assault of 10.1% for cis gay men and 9.5% for cis bisexual men in the past year [24], 39% lifetime contact sexual violence and 29.2% lifetime non-contact sexual violence for bisexual men and 17.7% and 33.3% for gay men [25], prevalence of SV reaching 31.64% in gay men and 29.44% in bisexual men [26]. Although all the studies mentioned above conclude that SV in the GBM population is drastically higher than in heterosexual cissexual men and similar to heterosexual cissexual women, and also that trans people have a higher risk of victimization, the figures differ greatly among them due to a lack of clear delimitation in the concept of sexual violence (e.g., sexual coercion, sexual aggression, unwanted relationships, intimate partner violence, etc.). It has been noted that while some studies define it very narrowly and only include some of its most obvious manifestations, others include a much wider range of situations [27].

There are a number of factors that indicate that the figures on SV may underrepresent the reality of this group. These factors are related to several barriers that affect GBM in relation to reporting experiences of SV. First, individuals who identify as male are particularly reluctant to admit psychological consequences that are inconsistent with male gender role expectations [28], resulting in poor communication of experiences. Such communication would actually be selective so they would need a higher level of distress to communicate such experiences [27]. In this sense, we should highlight the role of male socialization in understanding the differences in consequences and coping strategies between men and women when victimized [29]. Second, GBM are so stigmatized by their sexual orientation that they may encounter additional difficulties in communicating their experiences of SV for fear of further discrediting themselves [30]. It is also important to take into account the role played by how sexual relations and consent are conceptualized in this group since it is necessary for a SV situation to be labeled as such in order to communicate it in a relevant way. In fact, the most common method used by GBM to give consent is not to resist [31]. This makes it difficult to differentiate a consensual situation from a violent one, both for the perpetrator and the victim. There are some perspectives that claim that there is a "culture of silence" in the collective [32] that accepts, normalizes, and consequently obscures SV. Although it seems that some people in the GBM collective accept all these situations and do not cause them discomfort, some others are resisting such normalization [11], and they are having trouble labeling some experiences as sexual violence because they have them internalized. There are a number of factors that would result in an intentional ambiguity in defining what is and what is not SV in sexual minorities. Such factors would include stereotypes like gay men always want to have sex, gender norms regarding masculinity, a particular vision of queerness that could, in fact, foreclose the role of power dynamics, and the risk of social isolation when someone refuses sexualized social relations [33].

The aim of this study is to make SV visible for GBM individuals in Spain. To do so, the prevalence of victimization and the frequency in which certain specific violent situations occur, as well as some of their main characteristics have been studied. Emphasis has been placed on the communication of experiences; it is of interest to know to what extent victims communicate and to whom they turn in order to understand the low visibility of the problem and to propose preventive strategies and interventions. It is not the purpose of this study to pathologize the sexuality of men who have sex with men nor to suggest that violent behaviors are the primary framework from which we can generalize all GBM sexual experiences. Instead, it is intended to give voice to the discomfort experienced by some GBM individuals in order to promote a discourse that supports positive sexual experiences and the emotional well-being of GBM individuals.

2. Materials and Methods

2.1. Study Design and Data Collection

This is a cross-sectional study aimed at obtaining quantitative information through a self-administered questionnaire. Participation was anonymous and voluntary and aimed at the GBM population living in Spain. The final sample consisted of 550 respondents.

2.2. Measurement Tool

The questionnaire was built using Google Forms v0.8 software. The definition of SV from the WHO was used, through which SV situations were extracted and transformed into items [1]. Thus, the pilot version of the questionnaire consisted of these items.

It was administered for the first time in a small sample of GBM who had suffered some type of violence (10 participants) to ensure that there were no problems with the comprehension of the items and that the participants could give their opinions in general. Interviews were conducted with questions about the appropriateness of the items for the GBM collective in order to make them more sensitive to the reality of this particular group. Based on their recommendations, the questionnaire was reconstructed in such a way that new situations of sexual violence and more response possibilities were added to define their characteristics, as well as eliminating those questions that were labeled as uncomfortable or out of place. It was also decided to divide the experiences into two separate blocks (experiences with and without physical contact) to ensure that the mildest situations were asked first and that the most sensitive ones were presented little by little.

The final version of the instrument was intended not only to collect data but also to serve as a tool for participants to share their perceptions of the experience at length if they so wished. It can be seen as an attempt to provide a tool with which to express themselves, given the invisibility and problems inherent in communicating the experiences of SV in this group. The internal consistency of the questionnaire was $\alpha = 0.87$ for the total scale.

2.3. Variables

2.3.1. Socio-Demographic Information

Information on gender identity, sexual orientation, race/ethnicity, level of education to date and autonomous community of usual residence was collected. Questions on gender identity and sexual orientation were part of the exclusion criteria and sent some participants to the end of the questionnaire according to their answers. The responses referring to the autonomous community of habitual residence covered all those autonomous communities and cities that are part of the Spanish state.

To avoid bias, the questions that formed part of the exclusion criteria were asked before explaining the goals of the study and the target population. In this way, we tried to reduce the probability that participants who did not meet the admission criteria could falsify their identity, since once these variables were answered, participants were directed to the end of the questionnaire and could not participate again from the same email address.

2.3.2. Prevalence and Frequency of SV Experiences

To study the prevalence and frequency of perceived SV, participants were asked to what extent they have experienced a series of violent situations. The information about the frequency offers us not only information about what proportion of the sample has suffered each situation, but also informs us about the extent to which each participant has suffered those experiences. These frequencies were recorded on a Likert scale (1 = Never/2 = Once/3 = Sometimes/4 = Often/5 = Many times). Contrary to other studies, we avoided asking about the exact number of times each situation occurred. Firstly, it is difficult for participants to get the count of each situation right, especially when dealing with potentially traumatic experiences or almost normalized experiences. Secondly, because this study focuses on the victim's perception: a situation may have happened five times but for one person it may be labeled as "sometimes" and for another as "many times".

The blocks of experiences have been differentiated as done by other studies to allow comparison into unwanted insinuation, sexual coercion, and sexual assault. The situations that were part of unwanted insinuation were (1) Unwelcome sexually explicit comments (Comments) and (2) Inappropriate exhibition of genitalia (Exhibition). Sexual coercion included (3) Excessive insistence to have sex (Insistence), (4) Verbal recrimination (e.g., insults) motivated by the refusal to have sex with the perpetrator (Verbal Recrimination), (5) Blackmail and threats in order to convince the victim to have sex (Blackmail and Threats), (6) Physical punishment motivated by the refusal to have sex with the perpetrator (Physical Punishment), (7) Victim incapacitated (physically or mentally) to give consent or to resist (Self Incapacitation) and (8) Victim intentionally drugged by the perpetrator for sexual purposes (Chemical Submission). Sexual assault included (9) Unwanted touching with sexual intent (Touching), (10) Attempted rape: victim managed to escape the situation (Attempted rape), (11) Forced physically without penetration, whether oral, anal or vaginal (Forced without penetration) and (12) Forced physically with penetration, whether oral, anal or vaginal (Rape). Items (13) Intentional and unwanted injuries during sex (Injuries), (14) Image-based sexual violence: the perpetrator shows or posts sexual images of the victim without consent (Images) and (15) Refusal to use protection or not using it without the victim's consent (Protection) did not correspond to any of the previous blocks.

To avoid ambiguity to the greatest extent possible, the items have been written specifying that there must be a feeling of discomfort. In this way, an attempt has been made not to record those situations that were appropriate for the context. For example: "... without my consent", "... and I did not want it", "... and I think it was inappropriate".

If any participant answered "Never" in all situations, they were redirected to the end of the questionnaire because the rest of the questions were not applicable.

2.3.3. Situational Characteristics

Some information about the violent person has been examined. In order to keep the questionnaire brief, these characteristics have been recorded, as well as all of the following, for the overall situations of SV instead of asking for the characteristics of each of the situations separately. For this reason, it was reminded in these sections that in cases of having experienced several situations of violence or being protagonized by different perpetrators, the participant should mark all the relevant answers.

Regarding the age difference with the perpetrator, exact numbers were again avoided with the same justification: victims may have problems remembering all the exact ages (especially in cases where there are several abuses, several abusers or if he/she was incapacitated) and an age difference of five years, for example, may or may not be a clear age difference depending on the person and their relationship with the perpetrator. The gender identity of the perpetrator and the bond with the victim at the time of the abuse were also explored.

It was asked if any of the violent situations had been group aggressions and if any of them had been carried out by the same person more than once. Information about the place where the violent situation occurred was also collected.

2.3.4. Communication and Social Support

Participants were asked if they have shared their experiences, and if so, to whom they have shared them. A general question was asked about the potential usefulness of support groups (if they existed) for GBM individuals who have suffered violence. It was evaluated on a Likert scale (1 = Not useful at all/5 = Very useful).

2.4. Participants

The participants who were part of the sample met the following inclusion criteria: (1) identify as male (regardless of being cissexual or transsexual), (2) identify as homosexual or bisexual, and (3) live in an autonomous community or city in Spain on a regular basis. Any other answer to the questions related to gender identity, place of habitual residence or sexual orientation were discarded. Thus, if a total of 1220 responses were recorded, the initial sample included responses from the 690 participants who met the inclusion criteria. To ensure representation of the territorial distribution of the population, the number of participants from each autonomous community that was included in the study was proportional to the population of men in each community in relation to the Spanish total based on data from the National Institute of Statistics [34]. Thus, some responses from those autonomous communities and cities that were overrepresented were randomly discarded. The final sample that would later be analyzed was composed of the responses of 550 participants.

These participants were obtained from the dissemination of the questionnaire through social networks (Instagram and Twitter) with the help of various Spanish LGTBIQA+

associations and through a profile on Grindr, a dating application for GBM, which contained the link to the questionnaire.

3. Statistical Analysis

The statistical program Stata version 14.2 was used for data analysis. A univariate analysis has been conducted for the experiences of SV, situational characteristics and communication and social support. Bivariate analysis is meant to uncover the differences between sociodemographic groups regarding SV prevalence and frequency.

The responses to each situation of SV were interpreted dichotomously (1 = No; 2, 3, 4, 5 = Yes) for the prevalence study, following the criterion of "tolerance 0". That is, any violent situation was considered to be present if the participant responded with any value other than 1. Confidence of 95% was used for the elaboration of confidence intervals (CI) for the univariate analysis. Analysis of variance (ANOVA) was carried out to determine the differences between groups regarding experiences of SV according to their sociodemographic characteristics: gender identity, sexual orientation, age, race/ethnicity and educational level for the bivariate analysis. Statistical significance was interpreted with p-value < 0.05 from Student's t calculation. Bonferroni adjustment was calculated separately for the analysis of each group. It should be noted that some category values do not have a large enough sample size to generalize the results. Situational characteristics and social support were examined from a descriptive approach.

4. Ethics Considerations

The questionnaire construction and management considered the ethical aspects of the Code of Good Practice of the Autonomous University of Barcelona and the recommendations of the European Charter for Researchers, based on the fundamental principles of anonymity, freedom, honesty and responsibility. The participants were aware of the objectives of the study and gave their consent to participate in it.

5. Results

5.1. Sociodemographic Characteristics

Table 1 shows the sociodemographic characteristics of the participants who were part of the final sample. Most of them were cis homosexual white young men with a high educational level.

Table 1. Sociodemographic data of the participants.

Variables	n (%)
Sexual orientation	
Homosexual	413 (75.09%)
Bisexual	137 (24.91%)
Gender identity	
Cis man	538 (97.82%)
Trans man	12 (2.18%)
Educational level	
Higher education (University, CFGS)	432 (78.55%)
Post-compulsory secondary education (Bachillerato, CFGM)	81 (14.73%)
Secondary education (ESO)/No studies	24 (4.36%)
Special regime education	13 (2.36%)
Race/Ethnicity	
White	473 (86.00%)
Latino	65 (11.82%)
Bi- or multiracial	8 (1.45%)
Black	1 (0.18%)
Middle East	1 (0.18%)

Table 1. *Cont.*

Variables	n (%)
Age	
25–34	221 (40.18%)
18–24	191 (34.73%)
35–44	90 (16.36%)
45+	48 (8.73%)
Autonomous Community/City	
Andalucía	99 (18.03%)
Cataluña	90 (16.36%)
Comunidad de Madrid	77 (14.00%)
Comunidad Valenciana	59 (10.73%)
Galicia	31 (5.64%)
Castilla y León	28 (5.09%)
Islas Canarias	25 (4.55%)
País Vasco	25 (4.55%)
Castilla–La Mancha	24 (4.36%)
Región de Murcia	18 (3.27%)
Aragón	16 (2.91%)
Islas Baleares	14 (2.55%)
Extremadura	12 (2.18%)
Principado de Asturias	11 (2.00%)
Navarra	8 (1.45%)
Cantabria	7 (1.27%)
La Rioja	4 (0.73%)
Ceuta	1 (0.18%)
Melilla	1 (0.18%)

Note. The percentages on autonomous communities/cities differ a maximum of ±0.09% from the INE figures about male population.

5.2. Prevalence and Frequency of SV Experiences

Table 2 provides a summary of the prevalence and frequency of occurrence of each of the vs. items and blocks presented in this study. The most prevalent situations for the GBM group in Spain are unwanted insinuations (87.18–92.38%), especially consisting of explicit sexual comments that are inappropriate (83.80–89.61%). The figures on the denial of the use of protection (42.67–51.18%) are also relevant considering the great number of STDs in this collective. The prevalence of sexual assault (59.83–68.02%) is especially high, with a 54.30–62.70% prevalence of situations of unwanted touching. Figures on rape prevalence are also alarming, ranging from 16.57% to 23.40%. Results on frequency are coherent with those found in the prevalence analysis.

Table 2. Prevalence and frequency for each situation of SV.

VS Variable	Total Prevalence	[95% CI] Prevalence	Average Frequency	[95% CI] Frequency
Unwanted insinuation	90.00%	87.18–92.38%	3.01	2.91–3.10
Comments	86.91%	83.80–89.61%	3.07	2.98–3.16
Exhibition	76.91%	73.16–80.37%	2.95	2.83–3.06
Sexual coercion	87.27%	84.19–89.94%	1.78	1.72–1.83
Insistence	82.91%	79.50–85.96%	2.98	2.89–3.08
Verbal recrimination	58.91%	54.67–63.05%	2.17	2.07–2.27

Table 2. Cont.

VS Variable	Total Prevalence	[95% CI] Prevalence	Average Frequency	[95% CI] Frequency
Blackmail and threads	34.36%	30.39–38.50%	1.63	1.54–1.71
Self-incapacitation	31.09%	27.24–35.14%	1.54	1.46–1.61
Chemical submission	12.91%	10.22–16.00%	1.18	1.14–1.23
Physical punishment	10.00%	7.62–12.82%	1.16	1.11–1.20
Sexual assault	64.00%	59.83–68.02%	1.55	1.50–1.60
Touching	58.55%	54.30–62.70%	2.15	2.06–2.24
Attempted rape	27.27%	23.59–31.20%	1.38	1.32–1.44
Forced without penetration	23.81%	20.31–27.60%	1.36	1.30–1.42
Rape	19.82%	16.57–23.40%	1.30	1.24–1.36
Injuries	25.27%	21.69–29.12%	1.36	1.30–1.42
Images	25.64%	22.04–29.50%	1.47	1.39–1.55
Protection	46.91%	42.67–51.18%	1.86	1.77–1.95

Note. The blocks Unwanted insinuation, sexual coercion and sexual aggression have been calculated from the average of the items that comprise them.

5.3. Situational Characteristics

The results on the situation and characteristics of the perpetrator are presented below (Table 3). It is of interest to note that the perpetrator is a stranger to the victim in most cases (63.65%) and that their most usual characteristics are being a cis man (95.09%), older than the victim (68.96%) and online using gay dating apps (58.15%); 9.63% of the sample informs us to have experienced group violence and 29.86% to have experienced violent situations with the same perpetrator more than once. Most participants were victimized when they were 19–24 years old (58.94%).

Table 3. Situational characteristics of the SV experiences.

Variables	n (%)
Bond with the perpetrator	
Stranger	324 (63.65%)
Casual partner/date	173 (33.99%)
Acquaintance	146 (28.68%)
Friend	65 (12.77%)
Long-term relationship	41 (8.06%)
Ex-casual partner/date	25 (4.91%)
Family member	21 (4.13%)
Ex-long-term relationship	12 (2.36%)
Workmate	8 (1.57%)
Other	5 (0.98%)
Perpetrator age	
Older	351 (68.96%)
Similar ages	216 (42.44%)
Younger	33 (6.48%)
Don't know	20 (3.93%)

Table 3. Cont.

Variables	n (%)
Perpetrator gender identity	
Cis man	484 (95.09%)
Don't know	21 (4.13%)
Cis woman	12 (2.36%)
Trans woman	8 (1.57%)
Trans man	7 (1.38%)
Non-binary	4 (0.79%)
Group violence	
No	460 (90.37%)
Yes	49 (9.63%)
Recidivist violence	
No	357 (70.14%)
Yes	152 (29.86%)
Space/situation	
Online (dating applications)	296 (58.15%)
Perpetrators home	203 (39.88%)
Gay disco/bar	195 (38.31%)
Victims home	130 (25.54%)
In the street	107 (21.02%)
Online (other applications)	102 (20.04%)
Date	98 (19.25%)
Non-gay disco/bar	89 (17.49%)
Someone else's house	70 (13.75%)
Education center	24 (4.72%)
Other	12 (2.36%)
Victimization age	
19–24 years old	300 (58.94%)
16–18 years old	176 (34.58%)
25–34 years old	164 (32.22%)
Under 16 years old	83 (16.31%)
35–44 years old	45 (8.84%)
45+ years old	12 (2.36%)

Note. The sum of the percentages for each variable is in some cases >100% because participants could choose more than one response option.

5.4. Communication and Social Support

Finally, the responses regarding communication and social support are reflected in Table 4. The usefulness of the support groups for the participants was rated positively with a mean of 4.26 (95% CI: 4.17–4.36). Of all the participants of the study who have suffered any kind of violence, most of them did not share all their experiences (67.58%). Most of them trusted their friends to do so (84.48%).

5.5. Experiences of SV × Sociodemographic Characteristics

The bivariate analysis that has been conducted regarding SV experiences vs. Sociodemographic characteristics is shown below with the symbols * = p-value < 0.05, ** = p-value < 0.01, *** = p-value < 0.001.

In terms of prevalence, trans people report a higher prevalence than cis people in the situations of *Incapacitated* ** and *Rape* **, and in *Sexual Assault* *. Bisexuals also reported a higher prevalence than homosexuals in situations *Forced without penetration* *. The age variable had the greatest effect on the items referring to situations of SV, with the youngest respondents showing a significantly higher prevalence. This is the case for the items *Comments* ***, *Exhibition* *, *Insistence* ***, *Blackmail and threats* ***, *Verbal recrimination* ***, *Rape* *** and in the groupings *Unwanted insinuation* *** and *Sexual coercion* **. In addition, people with no studies or only compulsory secondary education have reported significant differences showing a higher prevalence of SV, in most cases compared to all other categories. This is the case for the items *Chemical Submission* *, *Injury* *, *Physical Punishment* *** and

Forced without penetration*. Finally, with respect to the Race/Ethnicity categories, differences were only found in the comparison between Latinos and whites, with Latinos reporting a higher prevalence of SV. Such differences are found in the variables *Chemical Submission ** and *Attempted Rape **.

Table 4. Communication and social support of the participants.

Variables	n (%)
Communication	
Yes, but not all situations	344 (67.58%)
Yes, all of them	109 (21.41%)
No, none of them	56 (11.00%)
Social support	
Friends	430 (84.48%)
Long-term relationship	120 (23.58%)
Mental health professional	77 (15.13%)
Brother/sister	46 (9.04%)
Mother	33 (6.48%)
Other family member	26 (5.11%)
Father	13 (2.55%)
Support group	13 (2.55%)
Teacher or similar	4 (0.79%)
Other	4 (0.79%)
Ex-long-term relationship	1 (0.20%)

Note. The sum of the percentages for each variable is in some cases >100% because participants could choose more than one response option.

Regarding the frequency of occurrence, the results are similar. Trans people reported higher frequencies in the item *Rape **. Bisexual people in the items *Forced without penetration ****. Younger participants in the items *Comments ****, *Exhibition ****, *Insistence ****, *Blackmail and Threats **, *Verbal Recrimination ***, *Rape **, the groupings *Unwanted Insinuation **** and *Sexual Coercion ***. People with no education or with compulsory secondary education in the items *Touching **, *Injuries **** and *Forced without penetration ***, the groupings *Sexual coercion *** and *Sexual assault ***. Finally, Latinos reported a higher frequency of *Chemical Submission **.

6. Discussion and limitations

First, it is necessary to review the characteristics of the sample to see how representative the results really are. Although it was intended to be representative of the Spanish territory, it is not representative of most sociodemographic issues, so some categories are underrepresented: the vast majority of participants were cissexual, homosexual, with a higher level of education, white and young. In this sense, the sample of trans men is particularly small, so the results should be interpreted with caution, although many articles agree that this group receives more violence than cis people [35]. The sample of people with special education and compulsory secondary education/no education is also insufficient, as well as those of all race/ethnicity categories except for white and Latino men. All of these difficulties were to be expected, since first of all, very large samples are required to do intersectional studies [36] and also, the GBM population is very much in the minority, so it is difficult to get participants, and consequently, to make it large and representative. Even so, the considerable sample size of this study is considered a strength for the reliability of the results for the GBM population in Spain.

Although one of the objectives of the questionnaire was to ensure its brevity, it would be much closer to reality to include non-exclusively categorical measures of sexual orientation and gender. Taking into account that from a constructivist perspective gender is constructed in each social interaction to the extent that heterosexist social conventions are repeated (or not) [37], it would be interesting to understand to what extent the tendency taken by this performance affects the directionality of the perpetration-victimization, rather than focusing exclusively on gender identity. Indeed, in that sense, the terms gay and lesbian, beyond signifying only preferences in the object of desire, could be well-recognizable social identities, perhaps authentic and proper genders [38]. There is a need to advance the study of gender from a non-categorical queer perspective in order to understand the phenomena studied in all scientific disciplines in a comprehensive way; specifically, in the field of SV. Exploring beyond a binary definition of gender could help to make violence against non-heterosexual individuals more visible.

Given the variability and multiplicity of definitions and interpretations of SV, we cannot assure construct validity in this study, although the items that form part of the questionnaire were elaborated on the basis of what the WHO defines as SV [1] and were modified under the evaluation of GBM individuals. The figures on the prevalence of SV in the group are extremely high, which is not surprising considering that a wide range of situations of greater or lesser severity have been examined and that this is a study on lifetime victimization. However, the numbers could have been magnified due to the method of data collection, as most participants have been recruited by a GBM dating app and may be more likely to have experienced SV situations than those who do not use them. Comparison with other studies is not possible, firstly because the instrument for exploring SV situations is different, but also because some studies have only focused on childhood or adulthood experiences, while others have only recorded situations that occurred during a period of time (usually during the 6 months or a year before participating in the study). In addition to all these differences, it is worth noting the different conceptions of the concept of SV or sexual assault [27]. The only studies with which comparisons could be made report a 54.0% [22] and 35.2% [39] lifetime prevalence of sexual assault, although the questionnaire they use is very different, the definition of sexual aggression is slightly different, and they are from different countries. Those figures are lower than the prevalence found in this study, which is around 64% for sexual assault. On the other hand, the study on frequency is quite atypical in a work of these characteristics, so there is no quantitative data with which to compare the results. However, it is consistent with the violent behaviors that have been labeled previously as normalized and that manifest themselves as unwanted sexual advances (comments, exhibition, insistence) and touching, which are precisely the variables that have shown the highest frequency averages (>2), as well as verbal recrimination [11].

Results show that bisexual men, transgender men, those with a low educational level, and Latinos are more at risk of experiencing SV. This fact could be related to the concept of homonormativity, which refers to the privileges that some LGTBIQA+ people have for conforming to heterosexual norms, so that those cis homosexual men, without disability, with normative bodies, gender expressions and affective relationships would get more social recognition, so those "deviant" people would be more vulnerable to suffer violence [40,41]. Still, the sociodemographic characteristic that most significantly affects victimization is age. In fact, it is curious that, as this is a lifetime victimization study, it is the youngest people who report the most violence in a very significant way. Although it is not possible from this study to establish causal relationships, it could be due to (1) generational differences in the prevalence of SV, probably due to the emergence of the internet and social networks or the existence of more nightlife spaces for GBM, (2) a greater ability to label violent situations correctly due to the influence of the fourth feminist wave [42] in younger people, with movements such as #MeToo or (3) a memory bias that would make it difficult for older people to remember violence in their youth, especially for mild experiences of SV.

Although the variable of victimization age, to our knowledge, has not been studied in SV within the collective, it has been studied in studies of intragender violence. The age variable is found to be the strongest and most consistent characteristic in relation to the victimization of any type of violence among gay male partners, a fact that they attribute to the acquisition of internal and external resources with age that are protective against violent situations [43]. However, in our results, it is much more frequent that the perpetrator is older than the victim. Considering that the majority of the sample in this study were young people, more studies are needed in the field of SV on GBM to determine whether age could be a power resource for the perpetration of violence against younger people.

In relation to spaces, the prevalence of SV in dating apps is particularly high. In reference to this, we should consider the manifestations of rape culture in such spaces, particularly through Grindr, the geolocation-based social network most used by men who have sex with men. It would manifest itself through violent comments and unsolicited nude photos, and extend beyond online interactions in the form of sexual assault, sexual coercion, and image-based sexual violence [44]. This is consistent with articles that emphasize how Grindr encourages its users to see each other as objects to be consumed and discarded at will [45], a fact that could be considered an ethical danger in that objectifying and instrumentalizing others for one's own sexual pleasure could result in avoidance and closure towards otherness [46]. The effects that this whole scenario may have on the reproduction of vs. is evident, as it produces sexual encounters in which pleasure is centered on oneself and not on the interaction between the participants, a fact that could hinder communication and the interpretation of consent signals. The data from this study invites us to rethink the design, structure and format of apps for encounters between men who have sex with men, inasmuch as it is one of the spaces in which most situations of SV occur. Also noteworthy is the prevalence of SV in nightclubs and gay bars, which could be explained by the effect that alcohol and other drugs have on the perpetration of violence by predisposed individuals [47], as well as on the vulnerability to victimization [48]. A study of the expectations of the people who frequent these spaces could be of interest in order to investigate the relationship they may have with the perpetration of violent situations.

Although several participants added in the "Other" option spaces such as saunas, chills, cruising areas, dark rooms, etc., they have not been addressed in this study because it would be too hasty to draw conclusions about SV from a quantitative point of view and could run the risk of stigmatizing these sexual practices. These are situations that could be understood as violent in and of themselves, which is why it is necessary to study them in-depth, from a qualitative framework, in order to investigate how consent operates in these contexts [49].

Almost all perpetrators, as reported by the victims, are cis males older than the victim. The bond with the perpetrator is one of the most interesting variables of the study, as it shows that the vast majority of violence is perpetrated by strangers. This implies that it does not make sense to study SV on GBM only in the area of intragender violence or intimate partner violence in homosexual relationships. The figures are very similar to those found in another study [21], especially high for strangers (33.3% vs. 63.65% in this study), casual partners/dates (29.40% vs. 33.99% in this study) and acquaintances (15.70% vs. 28.68% in this study). For future studies, it would be interesting to include more types of bonds, since the LGTBIQA+ group is very rich in forms of relationships (polyamorous relationships, exclusively sexual relationships, open relationships, etc.) and in this way, a representation closer to reality would be achieved.

Finally, the fact that the vast majority of victims communicate their experiences to friends rather than to other links refers to the phenomenon of *peers' communication* and is consistent with existing literature [16]. In that sense, victim support groups could be a useful tool to promote such communication.

It is important to note that all answers regarding situational characteristics and social support have been registered for all the situations of SV that the participants may have lived at once, so this study is not capable of attributing this data to any specific situation of SV. For example, we cannot tell from these figures if most rapes in particular are carried out by strangers or by acquaintances. Those difficulties were accepted to ensure the questionnaire's brevity, and therefore, to achieve the largest possible sample. As this is a preliminary study, it shows an overview of the problem and encourages other studies to further investigate the specific topics discussed above.

Although it is inevitable that the study presents a series of limitations, it is important to emphasize the importance of being a pioneer in the study of SV on GBM living in Spain, as well as its usefulness as a tool for communication and expression for the victims. It is necessary to promote the study of sexual violence in this collective, as it is for all the letters of the LGTBIQA+ group. Addressing this issue, and consequently constructing prevention and intervention strategies focused on the particularities of this collective, would have important positive health outcomes. Not only because it would improve physical well-being by preventing STDs and the physical harm a violent situation may involve, but because it would also have a positive impact on psychological well-being.

7. Conclusions

This paper reveals that sexual violence is common among gay and bisexual men. Findings show that prevalence figures depend on sociodemographic characteristics like gender identity, sexual orientation, race/ethnicity and educational level. Prevalence would also be higher in certain situations and spaces. Some of the perpetrators' and victims' most usual characteristics have also been examined. Furthermore, it has come to light that those who have been affected face challenges when it comes to sharing their experiences with others and that they mostly rely on their peers to do so.

Epidemiological research and interventions should take into account the intersections between gender identity and sexual orientation to better tailor prevention and treatment in this collective. Given the invisibility and stigma associated with this issue, this study highlights the usefulness that support groups could have in facilitating victims' communication. As a preliminary study, this paper could be useful for further in-depth research on the topics discussed above, such as sociodemographic factors related to the risk of victimization or the role of external situational characteristics to specific situations of sexual violence. It is necessary to promote the study of sexual violence in this group to understand the power dynamics that could underlie these situations.

Author Contributions: Conceptualization, X.C.; Data curation, X.C.; Formal analysis, X.C.; Investigation, X.C.; Methodology, X.C.; Supervision, L.M.C.; Writing—original draft, X.C.; Writing—review and editing, X.C. All authors have read and agreed to the published version of the manuscript.

Funding: This research received no external funding.

Institutional Review Board Statement: Not applicable. The protocol of the study was not evaluated by the Ethics Committee of our university because it did not include invasive procedures; it did not include collection, use, or storage of biological samples from subjects; nor did it include collection, use, or storage of genetic information from participants. Following the current Spanish legislation, approval from the Ethics Committee is mandatory only when a study protocol includes any of these procedures.

Informed Consent Statement: Informed consent was obtained from all subjects involved in the study.

Data Availability Statement: The data sets used and analyzed in the current study are available from the corresponding author on reasonable request.

Acknowledgments: The authors would like to thank all participants who have taken part in this study and all the LGTBIQA+ associations who helped with the dissemination of the questionnaire.

Conflicts of Interest: The authors declare no conflict of interest.

References

1. Krug, E.G.; Mercy, J.A.; Dahlberg, L.L.; Zwi, A.B. The world report on violence and health. *Lancet* **2002**, *360*, 1083–1088. [CrossRef]
2. Resick, P.A. The psychological impact of rape. *J. Interpers. Violence* **1993**, *8*, 223–255. [CrossRef]
3. Dobash, R.P.; Dobash, R.E.; Wilson, M.; Daly, M. The myth of sexual symmetry in marital violence. *Soc. Probl.* **1992**, *39*, 71–91. [CrossRef]
4. Schippers, M.; Sapp, E.G. Reading Pulp Fiction: Femininity and power in second and third wave feminist theory. *Fem. Theory* **2012**, *13*, 27–42. [CrossRef]
5. Cho, S.; Crenshaw, K.W.; McCall, L. Toward a field of intersectionality studies: Theory, applications, and praxis. *Signs J. Women Cult. Soc.* **2013**, *38*, 785–810. [CrossRef]

6. Crenshaw, K. Mapping the margins: Intersectionality, identity politics, and violence against women of color. *Stanf. Law Rev.* **1991**, *43*, 1241–1299. [CrossRef]
7. West, C. Partner abuse in ethnic minority and gay, lesbian bisexual, and transgender populations. *Partn. Abus.* **2012**, *3*, 336–357. [CrossRef]
8. Cohen, C. *Male Rape Is a Feminist Issue: Feminism, Governmentality and Male Rape*; Palgrave Macmillan London: Hampshire, UK, 2014; ISBN 978-0-230-22396-7.
9. Connell, R.W. Change among the gatekeepers: Men, masculinities, and gender equality in the global arena. *Signs J. Women Cult. Soc.* **2005**, *30*, 1801–1825. [CrossRef]
10. Struckerman-Johnson, C.; Struckerman-Johnson, D. Acceptance of male rape myths among college men and women. *Sex Roles* **1992**, *23*, 85–100. [CrossRef]
11. Gaspar, M.; Skakoon-Sparling, S.; Adam, B.D.; Brennan, D.J.; Lachowsky, N.J.; Cox, J.; Moore, D.; Hart, T.A.; Grace, D. "You're Gay, It's Just What Happens": Sexual Minority Men Recounting Experiences of Unwanted Sex in the Era of MeToo. *J. Sex Res.* **2021**, *58*, 1205–1214. [CrossRef]
12. Conrad, P.; Schneider, J.W. *Deviance and Medicalization: From Badness to Sickness*; Temple University Press: Philadelphia, PA, USA, 1992; ISBN 978-0877229995.
13. Adam, B.D. Neoliberalism, masculinity, and HIV risk. *Sex. Res. Soc. Policy* **2016**, *13*, 321–329. [CrossRef]
14. Brennan, D.J.; Bauer, G.R.; Bradley, K.; Tran, O.V. Methods used and topics addressed in quantitative health research on gay, bisexual and other men who have sex with men: A systematic review of the literature. *J. Homosex.* **2017**, *64*, 1519–1538. [CrossRef] [PubMed]
15. Finneran, C.; Stephenson, R. Intimate partner violence among men who have sex with men: A systematic review. *Trauma Violence Abus.* **2013**, *14*, 168–185. [CrossRef] [PubMed]
16. Freeland, R.; Goldenberg, T.; Stephenson, R. Perceptions of informal and formal coping strategies for intimate partner violence among gay and bisexual men. *Am. J. Men's Health* **2013**, *12*, 302–312. [CrossRef] [PubMed]
17. Wolff, N.; Shi, J.; Blitz, C.L.; Siegel, J. Understanding sexual victimization inside prisons: Factors that predict risk. *Criminol. Public Policy* **2007**, *6*, 535–564. [CrossRef]
18. Willis, D.G. Male-on-Male rape of an adult man: A case review and implications for interventions. *J. Am. Psychiatr. Nurses Assoc.* **2009**, *14*, 454–461. [CrossRef]
19. Ortega, A. Agresión en parejas homosexuales en España y Argentina: Prevalencias y heterosexismo. Ph.D. Thesis, Universidad Complutense de Madrid, Madrid, Spain, 2014.
20. ALDARTE. Centro de Atención a Gays, Lesbianas y Trans. Centro de Estudios y Documentación por Las Libertades Sexuales. Estudio Sobre Violencia Intragénero. Available online: https://www.aldarte.org/es/documentos-lanzadera.asp?id=174 (accessed on 7 April 2023).
21. Ratner, A.P.; Johnson, L.J.; Shoveller, A.J.; Chan, K.; Martindale, L.S.; Schilder, J.A.; Botnick, R.M.; Hogg, S.R. Non-consensual sex experienced by men who have sex with men: Prevalence and association with mental health. *Patient Educ. Couns.* **2002**, *49*, 67–74. [CrossRef]
22. Rosario, M.; Schrimshaw, E.W.; Hunter, J. A model of sexual risk behaviors among young gay and bisexual men: Longitudinal associations of mental health, substance abuse, sexual abuse, and the coming-out process. *AIDS Educ. Prev.* **2006**, *18*, 444–460. [CrossRef]
23. Edwards, K.M.; Sylaska, K.M.; Barry, J.E.; Moynihan, M.M.; Banyard, V.L.; Cohn, E.S.; Walsh, W.A.; Ward, S.K. Physical Dating Violence, Sexual Violence, and Unwanted Pursuit Victimization: A Comparison of Incidence Rates Among Sexual-Minority and Heterosexual College Students. *J. Interpers. Violence* **2015**, *30*, 580–600. [CrossRef]
24. Coulter, R.W.; Mair, C.; Miller, E.; Blosnich, J.R.; Matthews, D.D.; McCauley, H.L. Prevalence of past-year sexual assault victimization among undergraduate students: Exploring differences by and intersections of gender identity, sexual identity, and race/ethnicity. *Prev. Sci.* **2017**, *18*, 726–736. [CrossRef]
25. Chen, J.; Walters, M.L.; Gilbert, L.K.; Patel, N. Sexual violence, stalking and intimate partner violence by sexual orientation, United States. *Psychol. Violence* **2020**, *10*, 110–119. [CrossRef] [PubMed]
26. Wei, D.; Li, J.; Xu, H. Sexual violence among male sexual minority college students in Guangdong, China: A cross-sectional study. *Curr. Psychol.* **2022**, *in press*. [CrossRef]
27. Peterson, D.Z.; Voller, E.K.; Polusny, M.A.; Murdoch, M. Prevalence and consequences of adult sexual assault of men: Review of empirical findings and state of the literature. *Clin. Psychol. Rev.* **2011**, *31*, 1–24. [CrossRef] [PubMed]
28. Hensley, C.; Koscheski, M.; Tewksbury, R. Examining the characteristics of male sexual assault targets in a southern maximum-security prison. *J. Interpers. Violence* **2005**, *20*, 667–679. [CrossRef]
29. Javaid, A. The dark side of men: The nature of masculinity and its uneasy relationship with male rape. *J. Men's Stud.* **2015**, *23*, 271–292. [CrossRef]
30. Goffman, E.M. *Interaction Ritual: Essays on Face-to-Face Behavior*; Pantheon Books; Routledge: London, UK, 1967; ISBN 0-394-70631-5.
31. Beres, M.A.; Herold, E.; Maitland, S.B. Sexual consent behaviors in same-sex relationships. *Arch. Sex. Behav.* **2004**, *33*, 475–486. [CrossRef]

32. Segalov, M. Why Hasn't the Gay Community had a #MeToo Moment? The Guardian. Available online: https://www.theguardian.com/commentisfree/2018/mar/07/gay-community-metoo-moment-conversation-consent-sexual-assault (accessed on 14 February 2023).
33. Namaste, V.; Gaspar, M.; Lavoie, S.; McClelland, A.; Sims, E.; Tigchelaar, A.; Dietzel, C.; Drummond, J. Willed ambiguity: An exploratory study of sexual misconduct affecting sexual minority male university students in Canada. *Sexualities* **2021**, *24*, 1041–1060. [CrossRef]
34. INE. *Población por Comunidades Autónomas y Ciudades Autónomas y Sexo*; Instituto Nacional de Estadística: Madrid, Spain, 2019.
35. Stotzer, R.L. Violence against transgender people: A review of United States data. *Aggress. Violent Behav.* **2009**, *14*, 170–179. [CrossRef]
36. Bowleg, L. When Black + Lesbian + Woman ≠ Black Lesbian Woman: The Methodological Challenges of Qualitative and Quantitative Intersectionality Research. *Sex Roles* **2008**, *59*, 312–325. [CrossRef]
37. Butler, J. *El Género en Disputa: El Feminismo y la Subversión de la Identidad*; Muñoz, M.A., Ed.; Ediciones Paidós: Barcelona, Spain, 1990; ISBN 8449320305.
38. Bernini, L. *Las Teorías Queer: Una Introducción*; Editorial EGALES: Madrid, Spain, 2017.
39. Heidt, J.M.; Marx, B.P.; Gold, S.D. Sexual revictimization among sexual minorities: A preliminary study. *J. Trauma. Stress* **2005**, *18*, 533–540. [CrossRef]
40. Walker, A.M.; DeVito, M.A. "More gay' fits in better": Intracommunity Power Dynamics and Harms in Online LGBTQ+ Spaces. In Proceedings of the 2020 CHI Conference on Human Factors in Computing Systems, Honolulu, HI, USA, 25–30 April 2020. [CrossRef]
41. Scheuerman, M.K.; Branham, S.M.; Hamidi, F. Safe Spaces and Safe Places. *Proc. ACM Hum. Comput. Interact.* **2018**, *2*, 1–27. [CrossRef]
42. Cobo, R. La cuarta ola feminista y la violencia sexual. *Paradigma Rev. Univ. Cult.* **2019**, *22*, 134–138.
43. Greenwood, G.L.; Relf, M.V.; Huang, B.; Pollack, L.M.; Canchola, J.A.; Catania, J.A. Battering victimization among a probability-based sample of men who have sex with men. *Am. J. Public Health* **2002**, *92*, 1964–1969. [CrossRef] [PubMed]
44. Dietzel, C. "That's Straight-Up Rape Culture": Manifestations of Rape Culture on Grindr. In *The Emerald International Handbook of Technology-Facilitated Violence and Abuse*; Emerald Studies in Digital Crime, Technology and Social Harms; Emerald Publishing: Bingley, UK, 2021; pp. 351–368. [CrossRef]
45. McGlotten, S. *Virtual Intimacies: Media, Affect and Queer Sociality*; NYU Press: Albany, NY, USA, 2013; ISBN 9781438448787.
46. Dean, T. Unlimited intimacy. In *Unlimited Intimacy*; University of Chicago Press: Chicago, IL, USA, 2009; ISBN 9780226139395.
47. Abbey, A. Alcohol's role in sexual violence perpetration: Theoretical explanations, existing evidence and future directions. *Drug Alcohol Rev.* **2011**, *30*, 481–489. [CrossRef] [PubMed]
48. Kalichman, S.C.; Benotsch, E.; Rompa, D.; Gore-Felton, C.; Austin, J.; Webster, L.; Simpson, D. Unwanted sexual experiences and sexual risks in gay and bisexual men: Associations among revictimization, substance use, and psychiatric symptoms. *J. Sex Res.* **2001**, *38*, 1–9. [CrossRef]
49. Fernández-Dávila, P. ¿Se puede hablar realmente de actos de "violencia sexual" en los contextos de chemsex? Reflexiones desde los entendimientos de los hombres que practican ChemSex y la cultura sexual gay. *Health Addict.* **2021**, *21*, 124–137. [CrossRef]

Disclaimer/Publisher's Note: The statements, opinions and data contained in all publications are solely those of the individual author(s) and contributor(s) and not of MDPI and/or the editor(s). MDPI and/or the editor(s) disclaim responsibility for any injury to people or property resulting from any ideas, methods, instructions or products referred to in the content.

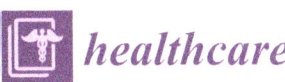

Article

Child Welfare Investigations of Exposure to Intimate Partner Violence Referred by Medical Professionals in Ontario: A Uniquely Vulnerable Population?

Nicolette Joh-Carnella *, Eliza Livingston, Jill Stoddart and Barbara Fallon

Factor-Inwentash Faculty of Social Work, University of Toronto, Toronto, ON M5S 1V4, Canada; eliza.livingston@utoronto.ca (E.L.); jill.stoddart@utoronto.ca (J.S.); barbara.fallon@utoronto.ca (B.F.)
* Correspondence: nicolette.joh.carnella@utoronto.ca

Abstract: Victims of intimate partner violence (IPV) and their children may be at an increased risk for negative health outcomes and may present to healthcare settings. The objective of the current study is to examine the profile of medical-referred child welfare investigations of exposure to IPV in Ontario, Canada. Data from the Ontario Incidence Study of Reported Child Abuse and Neglect 2018 were used. We compared medical-referred investigations with all other investigations of exposure to IPV. Descriptive and bivariate analyses as well as a logistic regression predicting transfers to ongoing services were conducted. Six percent of investigations of exposure to IPV conducted in Ontario in 2018 were referred by a medical source. Compared to other investigations of exposure to IPV, these investigations were more likely to involve younger children ($p = 0.005$), caregivers with mental health issues ($p < 0.001$) and few social supports ($p = 0.004$), and households noted to be overcrowded ($p = 0.001$). After controlling for clinical case characteristics, investigations of exposure to IPV referred by healthcare sources were 3.452 times as likely to be kept open for ongoing child welfare services compared to those referred by other sources (95% CI [2.024, 5.886]; $p < 0.001$). Children and their families who are identified in healthcare settings for concerns of exposure to IPV tend to receive extended child welfare intervention compared to those identified elsewhere. There is a clear difference in service provision in healthcare-originating investigations of exposure to IPV versus investigations originating from other sources. Further research into the services provided to victims of IPV and their children is needed.

Keywords: child welfare; intimate partner violence; healthcare; policy

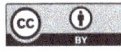

1. Introduction

In Canada, concerns regarding child well-being and safety can be reported to local child welfare agencies who determine the need for intervention. Studies have investigated the rate and characteristics of investigated child maltreatment in Canada at the national and provincial levels, allowing for the development of evidence-informed policies and practices [1].

Canadian child welfare systems frequently investigate concerns related to children's exposure to intimate partner violence (IPV) [1]. IPV, as defined by the World Health Organization, includes "any behaviour within an intimate relationship that causes physical, psychological or sexual harm to those in the relationship" [2]. Compared to other forms of investigated maltreatment (i.e., physical abuse, sexual abuse, neglect, and emotional maltreatment), exposure to IPV investigations comprise the largest proportion of substantiated child maltreatment investigations in Canada and Ontario [1,3]. The high rate of investigations of substantiated exposure to IPV is unique within the Canadian child welfare system; exposure to IPV is not a type of investigation that is routinely reported in Australian or American child welfare data [1]. Canadian studies have found that investigations of exposure to IPV tend to involve younger children, connection to support services that are external to child welfare, and substantiation of maltreatment without the provision of ongoing child welfare services or placement in out-of-home care [4–6]. It could be that child welfare represents an essential source of support and connection to necessary services for this vulnerable population. On the other hand, the tendency to substantiate exposure to IPV without the provision of ongoing child welfare services might suggest a limitation to the extent of support that child welfare can offer in these investigations.

Negative effects on children's mental and physical health associated with exposure to IPV have been reported [7–9]. As caregivers who experience IPV may also have negative health outcomes, including acute injuries, healthcare professionals represent important points of contact for children and families and need to be aware of the signs and how to screen for potential exposure to IPV [10,11]. Data from Ontario, Canada indicate that most child welfare investigations of exposure to IPV are the result of police reports, and therefore, reports by healthcare professionals represent a relatively understudied area [12].

Child welfare in Canada is legislated at the provincial/territorial levels [1]. In Ontario, child welfare services are mandated by the Child, Youth and Family Services Act [13]. Concerns of potential child maltreatment are directed to local Children's Aid Societies or Child and Family Service Agencies, which are funded by Ontario's Ministry of Children, Community and Social Services but operate as private non-profit organizations [3]. As defined by the Child, Youth and Family Services Act, there is a mandate in Ontario to report situations in which a child is at risk of or has suffered harm due to the actions or inactions of a caregiver [13]. While this legislation does not directly mandate the report of instances of an exposure to IPV, the assessment tool used in screening for child welfare investigations in the province, known as the Eligibility Spectrum, interprets this legislation to include violence between caregiver(s) or the child's caregiver and their partner [14]. Following a report to an Ontario child welfare organization, screening workers at the agency use the Eligibility Spectrum to determine whether the concerns meet the threshold to be opened for investigation.

In this study, we examine the profile of investigations of exposure to IPV referred to child welfare from healthcare settings. Our previous study examining the characteristics of child maltreatment-related investigations reported by healthcare professionals in Ontario found that 29% and 22% of investigations reported by hospital-based and community-based healthcare providers, respectively, involved a primary caregiver who was a victim of IPV [15]. Due to the physical and mental health impacts of IPV, caregivers and their children may require medical care, either in the emergency department or through primary care, depending on the urgency of their needs [11,16]. Previous studies demonstrate that victims of IPV utilize healthcare services more than those who have not experienced IPV [11,17,18]. It is estimated that there were over 10,000 emergency department visits related to domestic violence between 2012 and 2016 in Ontario, Canada [19]. Not only are victims of IPV more likely to access health services, but so are their children who may have been exposed to the violence [8,11,20–22].

Overall, it is well documented that there may be negative health consequences associated with being a victim of or being exposed to IPV. We are not aware of any studies to date that have looked at the profile of child welfare-involved families identified in healthcare settings for concerns of exposure to IPV or the child welfare response in these investigations. Our hypothesis is that medical-referred investigations of exposure to IPV will involve younger children and increased caregiver/household risk factors compared to investigations of exposure to IPV referred by other sources. We further expect medical-referred investigations of exposure to IPV to be more likely to be kept open for ongoing services given that the majority of investigations of exposure to IPV in Ontario are referred by police and tend to be substantiated without being transferred to ongoing services [6,12].

In order to test these hypotheses, our objective is to examine child maltreatment investigations of exposure to IPV in which the report of alleged child maltreatment came from a medical source. Data from the Ontario Incidence Study of Reported Child Abuse and Neglect 2018 (OIS-2018) are used. The medical referral sources captured in the OIS-2018 include hospital personnel, community physicians, and community health nurses. The specific research questions investigated in this study are the following:

1. What percentage of investigations of exposure to IPV were referred by medical personnel?
2. Compared to investigations of exposure to IPV referred by other sources, what is the profile of these investigations referred by medical sources?
3. Controlling for clinical and case characteristics, is a medical referral source associated with the provision of ongoing child welfare services in investigations of exposure to IPV?

2. Materials and Methods

2.1. Sampling and Weighting

Secondary analysis of data from the OIS-2018 was conducted to answer the research questions. The OIS-2018 is the sixth provincial-level study investigating the incidence of child maltreatment-related investigations carried out in Ontario, which is Canada's most populous province. Ethics approval for this study was obtained from the Health Sciences Research Ethics Board of the University of Toronto.

The OIS-2018 used a case review methodology in which child welfare workers provided information on investigations they conducted by completing online instruments. Investigations are the result of reports to child welfare organizations that meet the threshold for investigation based on the screening tool used in the province, the Eligibility Spectrum [10]. The OIS-2018 employed a multi-stage sampling design to obtain a representative sample of child welfare investigations conducted in Ontario in 2018. First, a sample of 18 (from a total 48) child welfare organizations in Ontario was selected for participation; consent for study participation was obtained at the organization level. The sampling period included investigations opened between 1 October and 31 December 2018. At larger agencies, the number of investigations included in the study was capped at 250. Lastly, participating workers identified children who were investigated for maltreatment-related concerns within selected cases. The final sample included 7590 child-maltreatment-related investigations involving children 0–17 years old in Ontario. These data were then weighted to provide an annualized provincial estimate. Please see [3] for a description of the study's weighting procedures. The final weighted estimate for the OIS-2018 was 158,476 investigations involving children 0–17 years old.

2.2. Data Collection Instrument

The online instrument completed by participating child welfare workers included three sections: (1) Intake Information, (2) Household Information, and (3) Child Information. The Intake Information section asked workers to include information on the referral, type of investigation conducted, and the household composition. The Household Information section included questions regarding caregivers living in the home, any potential household risk factors, previous child welfare investigations, transfers to ongoing services, and referrals to non-child-welfare-related services. The Child Information section collected information on child characteristics, forms and severity of maltreatment, and outcomes of investigations.

The OIS-2018 definition of child maltreatment-related investigations included investigations assessing allegations of maltreatment as well as those in which there were no specific allegations of maltreatment, but rather, the risk of future maltreatment for the child was being investigated. Where workers identified their investigation to be focused on allegations of potential maltreatment, they could indicate one of five primary forms of maltreatment: physical abuse, sexual abuse, neglect, emotional maltreatment, and exposure to IPV. Secondary and tertiary forms of maltreatment could also be noted.

The OIS-2018 data collection instrument asked about the individual(s) who made the report to the child welfare agency that resulted in the sampled investigation. The following referral sources were included in the OIS-2018: custodial parent, non-custodial parent, child, relative, neighbour/friend, social assistance worker, crisis service/shelter, community/recreation centre, hospital (any personnel), community health nurse, community physician, community mental health professional, school, other child welfare service, daycare centre, police, community agency, anonymous, and other. Multiple referral sources could be noted. In the present paper, we define medical-referred investigations as those with at least one referral from hospital personnel, a community health nurse, or a community physician.

2.3. Data Analysis

SPSS Statistics version 28 was used to conduct the present analysis. Using the weighted estimate of investigations of exposure to IPV, descriptive and bivariate statistics examining investigations referred by medical sources vs. other referral sources were conducted. Please see Table S1 for a summary of the variables used in the bivariate analyses. Chi-squared tests of significance were conducted using the sample weight for the OIS-2018. The sample weight weighs the estimate back down to the sample size in order to adjust for inflation of the chi-squared statistic due to the size of the estimate.

A logistic regression predicting transfers to ongoing child welfare services in investigations of exposure to IPV was conducted using the sample weight. Predictors were entered into the model in five blocks and were determined using chi-squared tests of significance, comparing various predictors with respect to transfers to ongoing services. The first block of the model included child ethnicity/race/Indigeneity and at least one functioning concern in the child noted by the investigating worker. The second block included the following caregiver risk factors: alcohol abuse, mental health issues, and few social supports. Household risk factors including overcrowding, two or more moves in the past year, and running out of money for basic necessities in the past six months were included in the third block. The fourth block included previous child welfare investigations and emotional harm noted to the child. The final block included our variable of interest, medical referral sources.

3. Results

Of the estimated 29,028 investigations of exposure to IPV captured in the OIS-2018 (10.82 investigations per 1000 children in Ontario), six percent (an estimated 1699 investigations; 0.63 investigations per 1000 children in Ontario) were referred by medical personnel (see Table 1). Table 2 compares investigations of exposure to IPV referred by medical professionals and all other referral sources according to the child, caregiver, household, and case characteristics. The medical-referred investigations of exposure to IPV involved younger children, with 43% of these investigations involving children 0–3 years old (compared to 25% of investigations of exposure to IPV referred by other sources; $p = 0.005$; see Table 2).

Table 1. Medical referral sources vs. all other referral sources in investigations of exposure to IPV in Ontario in 2018.

Referral Source	#	Rate per 1000	%
Medical referral source	1699	0.63	6%
All other referral sources	27,329	10.19	94%
Total investigations of exposure to IPV	29,028	10.82	100%

Based on unweighted sample of 1392 investigations of exposure to IPV.

Primary caregivers in investigations of exposure to IPV referred by medical professionals were more likely to have mental health issues identified by investigating workers (38% of these investigations) compared to investigations referred by other sources (22% of these investigations; $p < 0.001$; see Table 2). Primary caregivers in medical-referred investigations of exposure to IPV were also more likely to have few social supports noted by the investigating child welfare workers (34% of investigations referred by medical professionals vs. 21% of investigations referred by all other referral sources; $p = 0.004$; see Table 2). Ten percent of the investigations of exposure to IPV referred by medical professionals were noted to involve households that were assessed by the investigating child welfare workers to be overcrowded compared to three percent of all other investigations of exposure to IPV ($p = 0.001$; see Table 2).

Table 2. Characteristics of medical referral sources vs. all other referral sources in investigations of exposure to IPV in Ontario in 2018.

	Medical Referral Sources			Other Referral Sources			Total IPV Investigations			p-Value *
	#	Rate per 1000	%	#	Rate per 1000	%	#	Rate per 1000	%	
Child factors										
Age										0.005
0–3 years	724	0.27	43%	6781	2.53	25%	7506	2.80	26%	
4–7 years	372	0.14	22%	8025	2.99	29%	8397	3.13	29%	
8–11 years	340	0.13	20%	7321	2.73	27%	7661	2.86	26%	
12–17 years	262	0.10	15%	5201	1.94	19%	5463	2.04	19%	
										0.002
White	586	0.22	34%	13,623	5.08	50%	14,209	5.30	49%	
Black	306	0.11	18%	3631	1.35	13%	3937	1.47	14%	
Indigenous	133	0.05	8%	2566	0.96	9%	2699	1.01	9%	
Latin American	0	0.00	0%	1062	0.40	4%	1062	0.40	4%	
Other	673	0.25	40%	6447	2.40	24%	7120	2.65	25%	
Child functioning concerns								0.00	0%	
Developmental/physical	228	0.09	13%	2782	1.04	10%	3010	1.12	10%	0.327
Emotional	107	0.04	6%	2797	1.04	10%	2904	1.08	10%	0.237
Behavioural	121	0.05	7%	2093	0.78	8%	2215	0.83	8%	0.915
Primary caregiver factors										
Age										0.843
<22	-	-	3%	590	0.22	2%	639	0.24	2%	
>21	1650	0.62	97%	26,739	9.97	98%	28,389	10.59	98%	
Not cooperative/not contacted	-	-	3%	1721	0.64	6%	1777	0.66	6%	-
Alcohol abuse	-	-	5%	2935	1.09	11%	3025	1.13	10%	-
Drug abuse	178	0.07	10%	1784	0.67	7%	1961	0.73	7%	0.117
Mental health issues	640	0.24	38%	5895	2.20	22%	6536	2.44	23%	<0.001
Few social supports	576	0.21	34%	5636	2.10	21%	6211	2.32	21%	0.004
Household factors										
Income source										0.69
Full-time	885	0.33	52%	15,226	5.68	56%	16,112	6.01	56%	
Part-time	150	0.06	9%	3268	1.22	12%	3417	1.27	12%	
Other benefits	438	0.16	26%	5729	2.14	21%	6167	2.30	21%	
Unknown	-	-	5%	1273	0.47	5%	1363	0.51	5%	
None	136	0.05	8%	1832	0.68	7%	1968	0.73	7%	
2 or more moves in the past year	-	-	6%	1356	0.51	5%	1453	0.54	5%	-
Overcrowded home	170	0.06	10%	858	0.32	3%	1028	0.38	4%	0.001
Ran out of money for basic necessities in the past 6 months	135	0.05	8%	2893	1.08	11%	3027	1.13	10%	0.359
Child harm										
Emotional harm	136	0.05	8%	6581	2.45	24%	6718	2.51	23%	0.001
Physical harm	-	-	4%	221	0.08	1%	281	0.10	1%	-
Child welfare involvement										
Previous investigation	1045	0.39	62%	18,630	6.95	68%	19,675	7.34	68%	0.231
Substantiation	998	0.37	59%	16,551	6.17	61%	17,550	6.54	60%	0.713
Transfers to ongoing services	684	0.26	40%	6141	2.29	22%	6826	2.55	24%	<0.001
Referrals to services	874	0.33	51%	12,214	4.55	45%	13,088	4.88	45%	0.249
Out-of-home placement	-	-	4%	235	0.09	1%	302	0.11	1%	-

* p-value compares medical referrals and all other referral sources for investigations of exposure to IPV. —Estimate was <100 investigations. Based on unweighted sample of 1392 investigations of exposure to IPV.

Emotional harm to the child as a result of substantiated maltreatment was significantly less likely to be noted in investigations of exposure to IPV referred by medical personnel compared to all other investigations of exposure to IPV (noted in 8% of investigations of exposure to IPV referred by medical professionals and 24% of investigations of exposure to IPV referred by other sources; $p = 0.001$; see Table 2). Lastly, 40% of the investigations of exposure to IPV referred by medical professionals were kept open for ongoing child welfare services compared to only 22% of all other investigations of exposure to IPV ($p < 0.001$; see Table 2).

A logistic regression predicting transfers to ongoing child welfare services is presented in Table 3. As demonstrated in this table, various child (ethnicity/race/Indigeneity and at least one functioning concern), primary caregiver (noted alcohol abuse, mental health issues, and few social supports), household (overcrowding and running out of money for basic necessities), and case (emotional harm noted to the child) characteristics were significant predictors of the decision to transfer a case to ongoing services. After controlling for other variables in the model, investigations of exposure to IPV referred by medical professionals were significantly more likely to be transferred to ongoing services compared to all other investigations of exposure to IPV (odds ratio = 3.452; 95% CI [2.024, 5.886]; $p < 0.001$).

Table 3. Logistic regression predicting transfers to ongoing child welfare services in Ontario in 2018.

Variables	B	SE	p-Value	Odds Ratio	95% Confidence Interval	
Child Factors						
(White as reference)						
Black	−0.330	0.239	0.166	0.719	0.450	1.147
Indigenous	1.061	0.225	<0.001	2.890	1.858	4.495
Latin American	−0.751	0.482	0.119	0.472	0.183	1.213
Other	−0.606	0.198	0.002	0.546	0.370	0.804
At least one functioning concern	0.443	0.167	0.008	1.557	1.123	2.158
Primary Caregiver Factors						
Alcohol abuse	0.777	0.217	<0.001	2.175	1.422	3.326
Mental health issues	0.693	0.165	<0.001	2.001	1.448	2.765
Few social supports	0.488	0.168	0.004	1.629	1.172	2.266
Household Factors						
Overcrowding	0.841	0.337	0.012	2.319	1.199	4.485
2 or more moves in the past year	0.156	0.303	0.606	1.169	0.646	2.116
Ran out of money for basic necessities in the past 6 months *	0.512	0.222	0.021	1.669	1.080	2.580
Case factors						
Previous case openings	−0.044	0.165	0.790	0.957	0.693	1.322
Emotional harm	1.314	0.160	<0.001	3.722	2.718	5.097
Referral source (compared to all other referral sources)						
Medical referral source	1.239	0.272	<0.001	3.452	2.024	5.886

* Basic necessities include food, housing, utilities, telephone, transportation, and medical care.

4. Discussion

As a result of increased vulnerability to mental and physical health concerns for both children, who are exposed to violence, and their caregivers, who are victims of violence, children who are exposed to IPV may be more likely to come to the attention of medical professionals compared to their peers [8,11,20–22]. As such, medical professionals serve important roles in the identification of suspected exposure to IPV that may require child welfare intervention. The purpose of our study was to establish the proportion of investigations of exposure to IPV referred by medical sources, describe the profile of these investigations, and determine if medical referrals for investigations of exposure to IPV were associated with ongoing child welfare service provision when controlling for other factors.

4.1. Profile of Medical-Referred Investigations of Exposure to IPV

The results of our bivariate analyses indicate an increased proportion of certain risk factors in medical-referred investigations of exposure to IPV compared to those referred by other sources. Consistent with previous studies examining trends in hospital-based and medical referrals to child welfare agencies in Ontario, investigations of exposure to

IPV referred by medical personnel involved younger children [23] and were more likely to involve primary caregivers who were noted to struggle with mental health issues and few social supports [15]. These investigations were also more likely to involve households that were noted to be overcrowded.

4.2. Ongoing Child Welfare Services in Medical-Referred Investigations of Exposure to IPV

The results of our multivariate analysis reveal that, when controlling for clinical case characteristics, the investigations of exposure to IPV referred by healthcare professionals were nearly three and a half times as likely to be transferred to ongoing child welfare services compared to those referred by other sources (see Table 3). It could be that the increased vulnerability of this population (as evidenced by the young ages of the investigated children and the presence of certain caregiver and household risk factors) heightens child welfare workers' concerns for the overall well-being of these children. Therefore, these investigations are kept open to help establish more support for these families. Interestingly, these investigations were less likely to involve emotional harm to the child. This is, again, consistent with the workers keeping these investigations open to support the families and help to mitigate risk factors rather than to protect children from emotional harm as a result of exposure to IPV.

Previous work examining medical referrals for child-maltreatment-related concerns demonstrated that these investigations were more likely to be substantiated and involve more intrusive forms of child welfare involvement compared to investigations referred by other sources [15,23]. In a recent qualitative study examining the intersection of the child welfare and healthcare systems, child welfare workers reflected that this could be due to the perceived expertise and credibility of healthcare providers as well as the increased severity of cases referred by these sources [24]. Although there was no significant difference in the substantiation between medical-referred investigations of exposure to IPV and those referred by other sources, these reasons could contribute to the increased likelihood of investigations referred by medical personnel being transferred to ongoing services.

A study using data from the Canadian Incidence Study of Reported Child Abuse and Neglect 2003 documented a propensity for investigations of exposure to IPV to involve substantiated maltreatment but not be transferred for ongoing child welfare services or to be placed in out-of-home care [6]. More than half of the investigations of exposure to IPV in Ontario are referred by police [12]. Nikolova et al. [5] conducted interviews with representatives from police departments in Ontario to investigate the recent increase in investigations of exposure to IPV in the province. These representatives described a mandatory reporting policy requiring police to report all potential instances of exposure to verbal, emotional, or physical violence to child welfare agencies, even if the child is not physically present [5].

As previously mentioned, the screening tool used by child welfare agencies in the province, the Eligibility Spectrum, defines exposure to IPV as a reason for child welfare investigation. Therefore, police calls for exposure to IPV essentially automatically result in child welfare investigations. However, the police do not necessarily make these referrals based on clinical concern for the child, but rather due to the presence of a child. This is different from referrals by medical personnel where clinicians are likely making the decision to refer to child welfare based on the suspicion of risk or harm to the child. This could help to explain why investigations referred by medical personnel are more likely to be transferred to ongoing child welfare services.

4.3. Limitations

Several limitations should be considered when interpreting the findings of the current study. First, the data collected in the OIS-2018 are cross-sectional and represent child welfare workers' knowledge at the conclusion of their initial investigations. These data represent the clinical judgements of the workers and are not independently verified. As the OIS-2018 only captures investigations, child maltreatment cases that are not reported to child welfare, investigated only by police, or screened out prior to investigation are not included. Furthermore, no information regarding dispositions after the investigation stage of child welfare involvement is included. Three limitations to the weighting procedures should be noted. The correction applied to account for the agency size uses the overall service volume but does not consider the variation in investigation types across agencies. The annualization correction only accounts for seasonal fluctuations in the number of investigations but not the types of investigations conducted. Finally, cases that were re-opened within the same year are included in the annualization calculation, meaning multiple investigations of the same child can be counted. For this reason, child-level investigations is the unit of analysis of the OIS-2018 rather than investigated children.

5. Conclusions

Healthcare professionals are important points of contact for potential victims of IPV and their children who may be exposed to violence. Six percent of all investigation referrals to Ontario child welfare agencies for exposure to IPV originate from a healthcare source. Supporting our initial hypotheses, compared to investigations of exposure to IPV referred by other sources, medical-referred investigations were more likely to involve younger children and several caregiver and household risk factors, indicating a uniquely vulnerable population. Medical-referred child welfare investigations were also more likely to be kept open for ongoing child welfare services following the initial investigation. Postulated reasons for this include the aforementioned increased vulnerability of the children/families, perceived expertise of the healthcare professionals, or the nature of police-referred investigations, which represent the majority of investigations of exposure to IPV. Further research into the services provided to victims of IPV and their children, identified in healthcare settings, would help to elucidate how resources can be directed to identify and serve these families' needs.

Supplementary Materials: The following supporting information can be downloaded at: https://www.mdpi.com/article/10.3390/healthcare11182599/s1, Table S1: List of variables used in bivariate analyses.

Author Contributions: Conceptualization, B.F., N.J.-C. and J.S.; methodology, B.F.; validation, B.F.; formal analysis, N.J.-C. and B.F.; investigation, B.F. and N.J.-C.; resources, B.F.; data curation, B.F.; writing—original draft preparation, N.J.-C. and E.L.; writing—review and editing, B.F.; visualization, N.J.-C.; supervision, B.F.; project administration, B.F.; funding acquisition, B.F. All authors have read and agreed to the published version of the manuscript.

Funding: This research was funded by the Social Sciences and Humanities Research Council's Canada Research Chair in Child Welfare (#950-231186).

Institutional Review Board Statement: This study was approved by the Health Sciences Research Ethics Board of the University of Toronto (protocol code: #29325; date of approval: 29 May 2023).

Informed Consent Statement: Not applicable.

Data Availability Statement: The data are not publicly available due to confidentiality concerns and the sensitive nature of the data.

Conflicts of Interest: The authors declare no conflict of interest.

References

1. Fallon, B.; Joh-Carnella, N.; Trocmé, N.; Esposito, T.; Hélie, S.; Lefebvre, R. Major Findings from the Canadian Incidence Study of Reported Child Abuse and Neglect 2019. *Int. J. Child Malt.* **2022**, *5*, 1–17. [CrossRef]
2. Garcia-Moreno, C.; Guedes, A.; Knerr, W. *Understanding and Addressing Violence against Women*; World Health Organization: Geneva, Switzerland, 2012. Available online: https://apps.who.int/iris/bitstream/handle/10665/77432/WHO_RHR_12.36_eng.pdf (accessed on 28 June 2023).
3. Fallon, B.; Lefebvre, R.; Filippelli, J.; Joh-Carnella, N.; Trocmé, N.; Carradine, J.; Fluke, J. Major Findings from the Ontario Incidence Study of Reported Child Abuse and Neglect 2018. *Child Abuse Negl.* **2021**, *111*, 104778. [CrossRef] [PubMed]
4. Lefebvre, R.; Van Wert, M.; Black, T.; Fallon, B.; Trocmé, N. A Profile of Exposure to Intimate Partner Violence Investigations in the Canadian Child Welfare System: An Examination Using the 2008 Canadian Incidence Study of Reported Child Abuse

and Neglect (CIS-2008). *Int. J. Child Adolesc. Resil.* **2013**, *1*, 60–73. Available online: https://ijcar-rirea.ca/index.php/ijcar-rirea/article/view/73 (accessed on 28 June 2023).
5. Nikolova, K.; Fallon, B.; Black, T.; Passanha, N.; Isaac, K. Responding to Intimate Partner Violence (IPV) in Ontario, Canada: A Closer Look at Police Involvement. *Child. Youth Serv. Rev.* **2021**, *128*, 106168. [CrossRef]
6. Black, T.; Trocmé, N.; Fallon, B.; MacLaurin, B. The Canadian Child Welfare System Response to Exposure to Domestic Violence Investigations. *Child. Abuse Negl.* **2008**, *32*, 393–404. [CrossRef]
7. Nixon, K.L.; Tutty, L.M.; Weaver-Dunlop, G.; Walsh, C.A. Do Good Intentions Beget Good Policy? A Review of Child Protection Policies to Address Intimate Partner Violence. *Child. Youth Serv. Rev.* **2007**, *29*, 1469–1486. [CrossRef]
8. Holmes, M.R.; Berg, K.A.; Bender, A.E.; Evans, K.E.; Kobulsky, J.M.; Davis, A.P.; King, J.A. The Effect of Intimate Partner Violence on Children's Medical System Engagement and Physical Health: A Systematic Review. *J. Fam. Viol.* **2022**, *37*, 1221–1244. [CrossRef]
9. Grip, K.K.; Almqvist, K.; Axberg, U.; Broberg, A.G. Perceived Quality of Life and Health Complaints in Children Exposed to Intimate Partner Violence. *J. Fam. Viol.* **2014**, *29*, 681–692. [CrossRef]
10. Coker, A.L.; Davis, K.E.; Arias, I.; Desai, S.; Sanderson, M.; Brandt, H.M.; Smith, P.H. Physical and Mental Health Effects of Intimate Partner Violence for Men and Women. *AJPM* **2002**, *23*, 260–268. [CrossRef]
11. Rivara, F.P.; Anderson, M.L.; Fishman, P.; Bonomi, A.E.; Reid, R.J.; Carrell, D.; Thompson, R.S. Healthcare Utilization and Costs for Women with a History of Intimate Partner Violence. *AJPM* **2007**, *32*, 89–96. [CrossRef]
12. Fallon, B.; Black, T.; Nikolova, K.; Tarshis, S.; Baird, S. Child Welfare Investigations Involving Exposure to Intimate Partner Violence: Case and Worker Characteristics. *Int. J. Child. Adolesc. Resil.* **2014**, *2*, 71–76.
13. Child, Youth and Family Services Act, 2017. S.O., C.14, Sched 1. 2017. Available online: https://www.ontario.ca/laws/statute/17c14 (accessed on 28 June 2023).
14. Ontario Association of Children's Aid Society, Eligibility Spectrum. 2021. Available online: https://www.oacas.org/programs-and-resources/professional-resources/eligibility-spectrum/ (accessed on 28 June 2023).
15. Livingston, E.; Joh-Carnella, N.; Lindberg, D.M.; Vandermorris, A.; Smith, J.; Kagan-Cassidy, M.; Giokas, D.; Fallon, B. Characteristics of Child Welfare Investigations Reported by Healthcare Professionals in Ontario: Secondary Analysis of a Regional Database. *BMJPO* **2021**, *5*, e001167. [CrossRef] [PubMed]
16. Syed, S.; Gilbert, R.; Feder, G.; Howe, L.D.; Powell, C.; Howarth, E.; Deighton, J.; Lacey, R.E. Family Adversity and Health Characteristics Associated with Intimate Partner Violence in Children and Parents Presenting to Health Care: A Population-Based Birth Cohort Study in England. *Lancet Public Health* **2023**, *8*, e520–e534. [CrossRef]
17. Kothari, C.L.; Rohs, T.; Davidson, S.; Kothari, R.U.; Klein, C.; Koestner, A.; DeBoer, M.; Cox, R.; Kutzko, K. Emergency Department Visits and Injury Hospitalizations for Female and Male Victims and Perpetrators of Intimate Partner Violence. *Adv. Emerg. Med.* **2015**, *2015*, 502703. [CrossRef]
18. Gottlieb, A.S. Intimate Partner Violence: A Clinical Review of Screening and Intervention. *Womens Health* **2008**, *4*, 529–539. [CrossRef]
19. Singhal, S.; Orr, S.; Singh, H.; Shanmuganantha, M.; Manson, H. Domestic Violence and Abuse Related Emergency Room Visits in Ontario, Canada. *BMC Public Health* **2021**, *21*, 461. [CrossRef]
20. Schluter, P.J.; Paterson, J. Relating Intimate Partner Violence to Heath-Care Utilisation and Injuries among Pacific Children in Auckland: The Pacific Islands Families Study. *J. Paediatr. Child. Health* **2009**, *45*, 518–524. [CrossRef]
21. Bair-Merritt, M.H.; Feudtner, C.; Localio, A.R.; Feinstein, J.A.; Rubin, D.; Holmes, W.C. Health Care Use of Children Whose Female Caregivers Have Intimate Partner Violence Histories. *Arch. Pediatr. Adolesc. Med.* **2008**, *162*, 134. [CrossRef]
22. Casanueva, C.; Foshee, V.A.; Barth, R.P. Intimate Partner Violence as a Risk Factor for Children's Use of the Emergency Room and Injuries. *Child. Youth Serv. Rev.* **2005**, *27*, 1223–1242. [CrossRef]
23. Fallon, B.; Filippelli, J.; Joh-Carnella, N.; Miller, S.P.; Denburg, A. Trends in Investigations of Abuse or Neglect Referred by Hospital Personnel in Ontario. *BMJPO* **2019**, *3*, e000386. [CrossRef]
24. Joh-Carnella, N.; Livingston, E.; Kagan-Cassidy, M.; Vandermorris, A.; Smith, J.N.; Lindberg, D.M.; Fallon, B. Understanding the Roles of the Healthcare and Child Welfare Systems in Promoting the Safety and Well-Being of Children. *Front. Psychiatry* **2023**, *14*, 1195440. [CrossRef] [PubMed]

Disclaimer/Publisher's Note: The statements, opinions and data contained in all publications are solely those of the individual author(s) and contributor(s) and not of MDPI and/or the editor(s). MDPI and/or the editor(s) disclaim responsibility for any injury to people or property resulting from any ideas, methods, instructions or products referred to in the content.

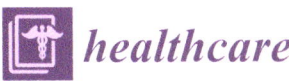

Article

Indicators Related to Marital Dissatisfaction

Claudia Sánchez [1] and Cecilia Mota [2,*]

[1] Coordination of Psychology Research, National Institute of Perinatology (INPer), Mexico City 11000, Mexico; clausanbra@yahoo.com
[2] National Institute of Perinatology, Research Tower, 1st Floor, Lomas Virreyes, Mexico City 11000, Mexico
* Correspondence: motaceci@hotmail.com; Tel.: +52-5555209900 (ext. 313 or 147)

Abstract: This is a study on indicators related to marital dissatisfaction. The research was conducted by the psychology department of a reproductive health institution in Mexico City. The objective was to know the relation between marital satisfaction/dissatisfaction and gender roles, self-esteem, the types of coping strategies and the types of violence perceived from the partner. It was a nonexperimental, retrospective, cross-sectional study of two samples—one of women and one of men—classified by marital satisfaction or dissatisfaction. The nonprobability quota sampling included 208 participants: 104 women and 104 men. Comparisons, correlations and a discriminant analysis were made to identify the most significant variables. Women with marital dissatisfaction perceived blackmail, psychological violence and humiliation/devaluation from their partner; they preferably adopt a submissive gender role and use escape/avoidance as a coping strategy, and so do the men with marital dissatisfaction, who also perceived blackmail, control and psychological violence from their partner; they have low self-esteem, and they preferably adopt a submissive gender role. Isolating factors will allow for more specificity in terms of psychological care at health institutions as well as avoiding gender biases and preventing an increase of violence in couples.

Keywords: marital dissatisfaction; intimate partner violence; self-esteem; coping; gender roles

1. Introduction

Marital satisfaction is related to behaviours that provide well-being and produce the ability to make agreements and solve problems in couple interactions [1–3]. In contrast, marital dissatisfaction has a negative impact on the quality of life, health and job satisfaction of people who live with it [4,5]; furthermore, it is a risk factor of domestic violence [6], which, to a greater extent, affects people who live in a couple relationship, their family and their surroundings [7–10].

Studies carried out in the Mexican population have indicated that both men and women believe couple relationships should be equitable for them to be satisfactory, and that they must communicate and solve their problems for the relationship to improve [11,12]. Other research on the topic has found several factors that are related to marital dissatisfaction; amidst the most noted ones are domestic violence, gender roles, low self-esteem and the types of coping.

The presence of domestic violence, defined as "an act or omission whose purpose is to hurt or wound another person, violating their rights" [13], p. 29, has been linked to a higher incidence of marital dissatisfaction in both women and men. Studies on heterosexual women show a high rate of psychological violence exerted by their partners, this being more frequent than physical violence [14], affecting their mental health and causing marital dissatisfaction [15]. Furthermore, it has been mentioned that domestic violence experienced mainly by women and girls has gone from being a hidden and tolerated event to a public health problem of a legal nature [13]; nevertheless, there are some studies that indicate that heterosexual men are also victims of violence by their partners, but it is less reported and has been made invisible due to cultural matters [16].

Gracia [17] noted that the reports of domestic violence show only a small percentage of the seriousness of this issue, with the added difficulty of it possibly turning into an actual lifestyle rather than being an isolated event. An example of this is shown in research on men who were victims of violence, where it was found that, due to the education they received and their social constructs, they did not have the ability to set boundaries, thus normalising the abuse exerted by their partner and creating marital dissatisfaction [18]. In this way, the presence of violence exerted by the woman towards her partner questions the notion that the woman is always the victim and that the man is always the abuser [19]. Likewise, a relation between other forms of violence—such as psychological violence—and marital dissatisfaction has been found [20–23]. In this regard, it is worth noting that psychological violence implies neglect, abandonment, infidelities, threats, insults, humiliations and the restriction of self-determination and decision-making power, all of which have an impact on self-esteem and produce feelings of deprecation and death wishes [24].

On the other hand, physical violence implies wounding the other person's body by means of physical strength with an object or weapon [8,24–27], which can last for years [28]. A study on Nigerian women experiencing marital dissatisfaction showed that physical and sexual violence exerted by their partners increased in those who had paid employment [29,30], whereas a similar study in the United States found that a decrease in pay gap reduces marital dissatisfaction and intimate partner violence [31].

Gender roles play an important part in couple relationships. Even when they are the product of socially established stereotypes for each gender [32], they may coexist in every person regardless of them being a man or a woman [33]. Furthermore, the distribution of both traditional and modern gender roles in a couple is influenced by their sociocultural context.

In contrast, the rigidity of gender roles in couple interaction increases marital dissatisfaction [11,34,35]. Shechory et al. [36] found that submissive women consider their marital life unequal, and they manifest poor sexual and marital satisfaction [37,38]. Likewise, Cazes [39] found that a patriarchal relationship still prevails in many couples in Mexico, where the woman must fulfil the traditional role assigned by society (maternity, house chores, etc.) even though the roles performed by both men and women have now evolved.

When diminished, self-esteem may also affect couple dynamics, producing marital dissatisfaction, for both women and men usually have self-deprecating responses [40]. Studies conducted in different populations have found relations between low self-esteem and marital dissatisfaction; for example, in violent Mexican indigenous women, a relationship has been found between low self-esteem and marital dissatisfaction [41]. Murray et al. [42] showed some differences in the perception of marital satisfaction between people with low self-esteem and people with high self-esteem. The former perceive that the issues in their relationship indicate a lack of affection towards them, causing them to respond with disdain and distance, thus generating dissatisfaction; on the other hand, the people with high self-esteem are less sensitive to problems and reaffirm their relationship by feeling satisfied. Another study where romantic relationships were analysed found a positive correlation between high self-esteem, happiness and couple satisfaction [43]. Aguilar et al. [44] compared the self-esteem of 48 abused women with 48 non-abused women and found that abused women show lower self-esteem than non-abused women, and that their relationships suffer from emotional abuse, impotence and hopelessness, all of which produce marital dissatisfaction.

Another factor related to marital dissatisfaction is the types of coping, which is a moderator between stressful events and the regulator of the emotional response to a problem [45–48]. It has been found that chronic stress appears when there is a lack of balance between the demands of the surroundings and the means to face them [49,50]. A study conducted in women with marital dissatisfaction and domestic violence revealed that the women with better coping strategies managed to better face this problem when compared to those who had less adaptive strategies [51]. Additionally, Puente-Martínez [52] compared the strategies of emotional regulation that were used by 200 women with marital dissatisfaction who survived intimate partner violence; the results indicated that they were passive at the beginning and used more active strategies later, which in turn helped them to end the abuse and dissatisfaction in their relationships.

Studying the factors that intervene in marital dissatisfaction and being able to isolate the variables that contribute to a better understanding of this interaction allows for the creation of more specific and efficient psychological intervention strategies.

Hence, the objective of this work was to study the relation between marital satisfaction/dissatisfaction, the type of violence perceived from a partner, gender roles, self-esteem and the types of coping used by a sample of Mexican women and men who visited a reproductive health institution to obtain indicators for a more specific psychological intervention.

2. Materials and Methods

A retrospective cross-sectional study with a multivariate, correlative, comparative design was conducted with two independent samples (one of women and one of men), each of them stratified according to the score they obtained on the scale for marital satisfaction/dissatisfaction, which was the classifying variable. It must be noted that the sample of men was selected by making sure there was an equivalence with the sample of women in terms of the control variables so both samples could have similar characteristics given that the subjects were not couples.

2.1. Participants

With an intentional nonprobability quota sampling, the samples were recorded during one year as stipulated in the project. The sample was composed of 208 participants, 104 women and 104 men, who entered the National Institute of Perinatology (Instituto Nacional de Perinatología, INPer) for medical care. The samples were recorded and analysed independently and not as couples. The inclusion criteria were: men and women of legal age, with minimum primary schooling, a one-year minimum relationship and no prior diagnosis of mental retardation or psychotic disorders. The controlled sociodemographic factors were: age, marital status, schooling (measured in years), occupation and the motive for visiting the INPer, which in the case of the women could be either obstetrical (pregnancy control) or gynaecological (any reproductive problem). As for the men, they did not have a medical diagnosis because they were only keeping a relative company who did have a medical appointment.

2.2. Procedure

The participants who met the inclusion criteria were given an identification sheet, and the application of the instruments was carried out in a single session before receiving any type of medical or psychological care. As part of their comprehensive treatment, psychological care was offered by the psychology department.

2.3. Ethical Aspects

The project was approved by the institutional research and ethics committees, with the following registration number: 212250-3110-10810-02-16. The participants signed the informed consent form, where it was specified that their data are anonymous and confidential.

2.4. Classification Variables

Sex and marital satisfaction or marital dissatisfaction.

2.5. Intervening Variables

Intimate partner violence, gender roles, self-esteem and types of coping.

2.6. Instruments

It must be noted that the psychometric indexes were taken from the original instruments that were validated for the Mexican population because, given the size of the sample, validations could not be conducted for the population of the study.

2.6.1. Multifaceted Inventory of Marital Satisfaction

It evaluates aspects of the couple's marital life with 85 Likert statements, validated for the Mexican population, with a Cronbach's alpha of 0.97 for internal consistency; the results were classified according to the scores obtained either above or below the cutoff point (188) [53].

2.6.2. Scale of Violence

It measures eight types of violence perceived in couples: physical, economic, intimidation, psychological, control, humiliation/deprecation, blackmail and sexual; it consists of 39 Likert test items validated for the Mexican population; the Cronbach's alpha for reliability was 0.97 [54].

2.6.3. Masculinity-Femininity Inventory (IMAFE)

It is a Likert scale that measures gender roles and is made of 15 test items per dimension (femininity, masculinity, machismo and submission). It is based on the most representative aspects of the gender roles and stereotypes found in Mexican culture. It was validated for the Mexican population, and the obtained Cronbach's alpha for reliability was 0.92 [55].

2.6.4. Coopersmith Self-Esteem Inventory (CSEI)

Validated for the Mexican population with a Cronbach's alpha of 0.81, it yielded two intervals: low level (less than 17) and normal level (18 to 23 points); it is made of 25 test items [56].

2.6.5. Coping Scale

It is made of 67 Likert test items and measures eight types of coping: Confrontational: direct actions to alter the situation; Distancing: efforts to remove oneself from the situation; Self-control: efforts to control feelings and actions; Social support: seeking support; Responsibility: acceptance of responsibility; Escape/avoidance: avoiding the problematic situation; Problem solving: efforts to change the situation with a reflective approach; Positive re-evaluation: creating a positive meaning based on personal resources. It was validated for the Mexican population with a Cronbach's alpha of 0.85. The highest score will be the ranking to be assigned [47,50,57].

2.7. Description of Samples

The final sample was made of four groups: women with and with no marital satisfaction (group 1 and group 2), and men with and with no marital satisfaction (group 3 and group 4). Measures of central tendency and dispersion were applied for the description of the controlled sociodemographic factors, and for the classification of marital satisfaction or dissatisfaction, x^2 and Student's t-test were applied. For the analysis of the variables, Student's t-test and Pearson's product-moment correlation test were applied. A discriminant analysis of the significant variables was performed to find the linear combination of the most significant variables to differentiate the groups. The analysis was performed with SPSS-22 software. The Student's t-test and the Pearson product-moment correlation test were applied to analyse the variables. A discriminant analysis of the significant variables was carried out to find the linear combination of the most significant variables to differentiate the groups. The analysis was conducted with the software SPSS-22.

2.8. Controlled Sociodemographic Factors

The characteristics of the samples, where some of the participants were a couple, were captured and worked on independently; however, this contributed to the similarity of the samples, which are shown in Table 1.

Table 1. Characteristics of the sociodemographic factors of the samples.

Variables	Women n = 104	Men n = 104
Age	32.3 ± 6.14 Range: 22 to 56 years old	35.1 ± 8.04 Range: 22 to 59 years old
Schooling	12.3 ± 3.23 years	13.0 ± 3.58 years
Married	64 (61.5%)	64 (61.5%)
Single	1 (1%)	6 (3.4%)
Civil union	39 (37.5%)	39 (37.5%)
Obstetrical	40 (38.5%)	40 (38.5%)
Gynaecological	64 (61.6%)	64 (61.6%)
Relationship/partner average	7.1 ± 5.2	7.1 ± 5.2

Regarding occupation, women were distributed as follows: 77.9% (81) were housewives, 8.7% (9) were employees, 7.7% (8) were underemployed (informal jobs) and 5.8% (6) were professionals (they practise a specialised academic profession). In men, the distribution was as follows: 58.7% (61) were employees, 28.8% (30) were underemployed and 12.5% (13) were professionals.

3. Results

Regarding the classification of marital satisfaction and marital dissatisfaction in the group of 104 women, 43 (41.3%) reported being satisfied in their relationship (group 1), and 61 (58.7%) expressed being unsatisfied (group 2). In the group of men, 58 (55.8%) reported being satisfied (group 3), whereas 46 (44.2%) said they were not (group 4) (see Table 2).

Table 2. Differences between marital satisfaction and dissatisfaction by gender.

	With Marital Satisfaction	With Marital Dissatisfaction	Total	x^2	p
Women	43 (41.3%)	61 (58.7%)	104		
Men	58 (55.8%)	46 (44.2%)	104	4.33	0.05 *

* $p \leq 0.05$.

Regarding the results through the *t*-test between women and men with marital satisfaction, women presented significantly lower scores than men (see Table 3).

Table 3. Comparison between marital satisfaction and dissatisfaction by gender.

	Marital Satisfaction n = 104 Mean DS	*t* value	Sig.
Women	3.87 ± 0.66	2.201	0.02 **
Men	4.06 ± 0.56		

** $p \leq 0.01$.

In the results of the study variables classified by gender and by marital satisfaction or dissatisfaction, the following results were obtained.

In women, statistically significant differences were found between those satisfied (group 1) and those unsatisfied (group 2) in terms of gender dimensions: femininity, masculinity and submission. Femininity and masculinity turned out to be related to marital satisfaction, whereas submission was related to dissatisfaction. Regarding self-esteem, statistically significant differences were also observed between groups 1 and 2, with higher scores found in group 1.

As for the types of coping, significant differences between group 1 and group 2 were only found in escape/avoidance, which was related to marital dissatisfaction. Problem solving and positive re-evaluation were related to marital satisfaction in spite of their marginal significance (see Table 4).

Table 4. Differences and relation between women with and with no marital satisfaction and their gender role, self-esteem and type of coping.

	Group 1 with Marital Satisfaction n = 43 Mean SD	Group 2 with Marital Dissatisfaction n = 61 Mean SD	t Value	Sig.	η
Femininity	5.48 ± 0.97	4.77 ± 0.99	3.63	0.000 ***	0.34
Masculinity	4.69 ± 0.88	4.23 ± 0.92	2.57	0.012 **	0.24
Machismo	2.90 ± 0.85	3.20 ± 0.93	−1.68	0.09	
Submission	2.37 ± 0.65	2.87 ± 0.77	−3.41	0.001 ***	−0.33
Self-esteem	19.3 ± 4.14	15.9 ± 5.23	3.70	0.000 ***	0.33
Confrontational	10.4 ± 2.63	9.9 ± 2.92	0.795	0.429	
Distancing	8.8 ± 3.04	8.02 ± 2.80	1.45	0.148	
Self-control	9.3 ± 2.85	10.1 ± 2.82	−1.28	0.201	
Social support	11.6 ± 3.19	10.6 ± 3.82	1.40	0.163	
Responsibility	6.5 ± 2.47	6.8 ± 2.70	−0.585	0.560	
Escape/avoidance	6.0 ± 3.62	8.8 ± 4.24	−3.45	0.001 ***	−0.33
Problem solving	11.8 ± 2.64	10.7 ± 3.30	1.91	0.059 *	0.18
Positive re-evaluation	14.4 ± 3.83	12.6 ± 3.8	2.35	0.020 *	0.22

* $p \leq 0.05$, ** $p \leq 0.01$, *** $p \leq 0.001$.

Furthermore, in terms of the types of violence, significant differences between group 1 and group 2 were found for all types of violence in relation to marital dissatisfaction with the exception of physical violence (see Table 5). It must be noted that the effect sizes in the significant variables went from low to medium.

Table 5. Differences and relation between women with and with no marital satisfaction and the types of violence perceived in their partner.

Types of Violence	Group 1 with Marital Satisfaction n = 43 Mean SD	Group 2 with Marital Dissatisfaction n = 61 Mean SD	t Value	Sig.	η
Physical	1.00 ± 0.00	1.03 ± 0.12	−1.91	0.060	
Economic	1.12 ± 0.28	1.55 ± 0.75	−4.04	0.000 ***	−0.35
Intimidation	1.04 ± 0.15	1.32 ± 0.57	−3.55	0.001 ***	−0.31
Psychological	1.09 ± 0.19	1.63 ± 0.86	−4.70	0.000 ***	−0.39
Control	1.17 ± 0.40	1.61 ± 0.93	−3.29	0.001 ***	−0.29
Humiliation/devaluation	1.01 ± 0.15	1.40 ± 0.65	−4.36	0.000 ***	−0.38
Blackmail	1.05 ± 0.10	1.58 ± 0.68	−5.97	0.000 ***	−0.47
Sexual	1.10 ± 0.23	1.41 ± 0.69	−3.29	0.002 ***	−0.28

*** $p \leq 0.001$.

In the sample of men, statistically significant differences were observed between those who were maritally satisfied (group 3) and those who were not (group 4) in terms of gender dimensions: femininity was related to satisfaction, and machismo and submission were related to dissatisfaction (see Table 6).

Table 6. Differences and relation between men with and with no marital satisfaction and their gender role, self-esteem and type of coping.

	Group 3 with Marital Satisfaction n = 58 Mean SD	Group 4 with Marital Dissatisfaction n = 46 Mean SD	t Value	Sig.	η
Femininity	5.24 ± 0.83	4.75 ± 1.01	2.70	0.008 **	0.25
Masculinity	5.01 ± 0.77	4.85 ± 0.94	0.892	0.375	
Machismo	2.84 ± 0.81	3.40 ± 0.88	−3.37	0.001 **	−0.31
Submission	2.31 ± 0.66	2.72 ± 0.86	−2.75	0.007 **	−0.25
Self-esteem	21.0 ± 2.60	17.2 ± 4.62	4.99	0.000 ***	0.45
Confrontational	10.3 ± 2.97	10.3 ± 3.11	0.010	0.992	
Distancing	8.0 ± 2.92	8.4 ± 3.26	−0.687	0.494	
Self-control	11.0 ± 2.97	11.2 ± 3.85	−0.390	0.697	
Social support	10.8 ± 2.91	10.4 ± 3.56	0.625	0.533	
Responsibility	6.6 ± 1.90	6.7 ± 1.98	−0.241	0.810	
Escape/avoidance	5.0 ± 3.37	7.0 ± 3.96	−2.89	0.005 ***	0.54
Problem solving	13.1 ± 2.74	11.8 ± 3.07	2.29	0.024 *	0.44
Positive re-evaluation	14.0 ± 3.26	13.3 ± 4.04	0.983	0.328	

* $p \leq 0.05$, ** $p \leq 0.01$, *** $p \leq 0.001$.

The high self-esteem scores were also related to satisfaction, and, regarding the types of coping, escape/avoidance turned out to be related to dissatisfaction, while problem-solving was related to marital satisfaction (see Table 6). As for the types of violence, statistically significant differences were also found between groups 3 and 4, with all the types of perceived violence being related to marital dissatisfaction (see Table 7). The effect size in men was medium.

Table 7. Differences and relation between men with and with no marital satisfaction and the types of violence perceived in their partner.

Types of Violence	Group 3 with Marital Satisfaction n = 58 Mean SD	Group 4 with Marital Dissatisfaction n = 46 Mean SD	t Value	Sig.	η
Physical	1.10 ± 0.05	1.17 ± 0.52	−2.16	0.036 *	−0.09
Economic	1.22 ± 0.42	1.83 ± 0.87	−4.29	0.000 *	−0.40
Intimidation	1.06 ± 0.18	1.45 ± 0.75	−3.37	0.001 ***	−0.33
Psychological	1.23 ± 0.45	1.84 ± 0.78	−4.67	0.000 ***	−0.43
Control	1.25 ± 0.40	2.23 ± 1.03	−6.07	0.000 ***	−0.53
Humiliation-devaluation	1.11 ± 0.26	1.57 ± 0.77	−3.83	0.000 ***	−0.37
Blackmail	1.12 ± 0.28	1.76 ± 0.78	−5.29	0.000 ***	−0.47
Sexual	1.09 ± 0.22	1.48 ± 0.71	−3.65	0.001 ***	−0.34

* $p \leq 0.05$, *** $p \leq 0.001$.

Correlations were made in both women and men between the studied variables and marital satisfaction/dissatisfaction with the purpose of identifying the most significant variables (Tables 8 and 9).

The discriminant analysis was performed with the significant variables in women and men. For the women, a function with 13 variables was obtained, explaining 100% of the differences and the variance between satisfied and unsatisfied women, an eigenvalue of 0.611, a Wilks' lambda of 0.621, and a canonical correlation of 0.616 with a significance of $p \leq 0.001$, which allowed the discrimination of the variables related to marital satisfaction or dissatisfaction. The standardised coefficients showed that violence is the variable that most contributes to marital dissatisfaction, particularly that of blackmail (0.639); it is followed by psychological violence, humiliation/devaluation, economic violence (controlling someone through money), intimidation, control and sexual violence; they preferably settle for a submissive gender role and use escape-avoidance as coping. By contrast, women with marital satisfaction showed an adequate level of self-esteem, a preference for feminine or masculine gender roles, and positive re-evaluation as their type of coping. The centroids showed −0.922 for satisfied women and 0.650 for unsatisfied women. Therefore, it can be concluded that women with and with no marital satisfaction have specific indicators related to this condition in 76.0% of the correctly classified cases; see Table 10.

Table 8. Correlations between the studied variables and marital satisfaction in women.

Variable	Marital Satisfaction r
Gender role	
Femininity	0.338 **
Masculinity	0.247 *
Machismo	0.164
Submission	−0.320 **
Self-esteem	0.333 **
Coping Style	
Confrontational	0.078
Distancing	0.143
Self-control	−0.126
Social support	0.138
Responsibility	−0.058
Escape/avoidance	−0.323 **
Problem solving	0.186
Positive re-evaluation	0.227 *
Types of violence	
Physical	−0.157
Economic	−0.332 **
Intimidation	0.290 **
Psychological	−0.370 **
Control	−0.278 **
Humiliation/devaluation	−0.346 **
Blackmail	−0.447 **
Sexual	−0.266 **

* $p \leq 0.05$, ** $p \leq 0.01$.

Table 9. Correlations between the studied variables and marital satisfaction in men.

Variable	Marital Satisfaction r
Gender role	
Femininity	0.259 **
Masculinity	0.090
Machismo	−0.317 **
Submission	−0.263 **
Self-esteem	0.465 **
Coping	
Confrontational	0.001
Distancing	−0.068
Self-control	−0.039
Social support	0.062
Responsibility	−0.024
Escape/avoidance	−0.276 **
Problem solving	0.221 *
Positive re-evaluation	0.097

Table 9. Cont.

Variable	Marital Satisfaction r
Type of violence	
Physical	−0.234 *
Economic	−0.415 **
Intimidation	−0.347 **
Psychological	−0.441 **
Control	−0.548 **
Humiliation/devaluation	−0.384 **
Blackmail	−0.498 **
Sexual	−0.371 **

* $p \leq 0.05$, ** $p \leq 0.01$.

Table 10. Structure matrix of the discriminant canonical functions: Women.

	Function 1
V Blackmail	0.639
V Psychological	0.509
V Humiliation-devaluation	0.472
Femininity	−0.460
Self-esteem	−0.451
V Economic	0.450
Escape-avoidance	0.437
Submission	0.433
V Intimidation	0.387
V Control	0.370
V Sexual	0.353
Masculinity	−0.325
Positive revaluation	−0.298

For the men, the discriminant analysis was performed with the significant variables; a function with 13 variables was obtained, explaining 100% of the differences and the variance between satisfied and unsatisfied men, an eigenvalue of 0.808, a Wilks' lambda of 0.553, and a canonical correlation of 0.669 with a significance of $p \leq 0.001$, which allowed the discrimination of the variables related to marital satisfaction or dissatisfaction. The standardised coefficients showed that men with marital dissatisfaction perceive control-type violence from their partner, which is the variable that most contributes to marital dissatisfaction with 0.728; it is followed by blackmail, psychological violence, economic violence, humiliation/devaluation, sexual violence, intimidation and physical violence; they preferably settle for a submissive gender role and use escape/avoidance as coping. By contrast, men with marital satisfaction showed an adequate level of self-esteem, a preference for feminine gender roles, and problem solving as their type of coping. The centroids showed -.793 for satisfied men, and 1.000 for unsatisfied men. Hence, it can be concluded that men with marital dissatisfaction have specific indicators related to this condition in 84.6% of the correctly classified cases (see Table 11).

Table 11. Structure matrix of the discriminant canonical functions: Men.

	Function 1
V Control	0.728
V Blackmail	0.638
Self-esteem	−0.585
V Psychological	0.546
V Economic	0.508
V Humiliation/devaluation	0.463

Table 11. *Cont.*

	Function 1
V Sexual	0.444
V Intimidation	0.412
Escape/avoidance	0.319
Submission	0.303
Femininity	−0.298
V Physical	0.267
Problem solving	−0.252

4. Discussion

The objective of this paper was to study the relation between marital satisfaction/dissatisfaction, the type of perceived violence, gender roles, self-esteem and coping styles in a sample of Mexican women and men. One of the early findings was the differences between women and men in terms of the percentages for marital satisfaction/dissatisfaction; the percentage of unsatisfied women is 14.5% greater than that of unsatisfied men, which shows a disadvantage for women.

A second finding was the indicators associated to both marital satisfaction and dissatisfaction. Regarding those related to marital dissatisfaction, some similarities were found between both sexes.

The first indicator associated to marital dissatisfaction in both women and men was the perceived violence; the difference lies in the type of violence exerted on the other. In women, the most important factor was perceiving blackmail from their partner, followed by psychological abuse and humiliation/devaluation; in men, it was the perception of their partner exerting control over them, followed by blackmail, psychological and economic abuse. This coincides with Moral et al. [58], who stated that when conflicts are faced inadequately, these become chronic, leading to fights, distancing, indifference and, finally, to violence.

These results differ from what has been noted by other research carried out in Mexico where women are emphasized as the victims of marital violence [59,60]. Possibly, the difference between results is due to the way people tend to give socially desirable answers marked by gender prejudices in massive surveys. Nevertheless, couple violence has been studied in other Latin American countries where similar results to the ones obtained in this study have been found [61].

This would indicate that it cannot be stated that the man is the only one exerting violence in a couple, for many of these examples of violence are focused on the woman as the victim of the man [23,62,63]; therefore, it is important to do research with both sexes to widen the scope of the problem.

However, it must be noted that the studied population for this research comes from the general Mexican population because the INPer is not an institution specialised in women who were victims of violence with a prevalence of physical violence, where different factors could be found.

The second indicator related to marital dissatisfaction has to do with the gender roles established by couple dynamics; the results showed that submission prevailed as a characteristic in both maritally unsatisfied women and men. This coincides with a study on women and the relation between emotional dependency and intimate partner violence, where a high relation was found between the presence of both conditions in couples, resulting in attitudes of subordination and submission [64].

Low self-esteem was the third indicator found in women and men with marital dissatisfaction, which coincides with Echeburúa [65], who found that men with low self-esteem felt unsatisfied in their relationship and showed high levels of jealousy, possessiveness, irritability towards boundaries and poor impulse control. People with low self-esteem frequently struggle with self-confidence; when it comes to marriage, this insecurity leads them to behave in a way that fosters distancing, violence and dissatisfaction instead of contributing to a satisfactory couple dynamic.

The escape/avoidance type of coping was the fourth indicator related to marital dissatisfaction in both women and men; it is translated as avoiding conflict. Méndez and García [66] also found that this type of coping is a variable that predicts several types of violence that generate dissatisfaction in a relationship. This behaviour emphasizes marital dissatisfaction because it prevents both partners from facing conflicts and modifying some of their elements. Behaviours such as indifference, the silent treatment and not taking any actions to solve problems contribute to dissatisfaction, and they are risk factors that lead to violence [67].

In contrast, the first indicator related to marital satisfaction in both women and men was high levels of self-esteem. Our results showed that women and men who scored high levels of marital satisfaction also had high self-esteem.

A possible explanation for this is that people who trust their abilities and have a positive image of themselves are able to establish effective communication with their partner, express their needs and wishes in a clear way, and set healthy boundaries. They also tend to be less critical of themselves and their partner, which helps to avoid unnecessary conflicts [68].

In second place, we found that marital satisfaction is related to femininity and masculinity in women, for they involve demonstrations of affection and the care for others as well as self-affirmation. Likewise, in maritally satisfied men, femininity was the one prevailing characteristic.

The last indicator related to marital satisfaction in women was positive re-evaluation as a type of coping, which is a strategy centred on the control of emotion when facing a stressful situation, giving it a positive meaning that functions as an adaptive resource. In men, the prevailing type of coping was that of problem-solving, which consists of making an effort to change a stressful situation by means of reflection and assertive behaviour.

The found indicators allow us to better steer the psychological intervention as referenced by Santelices [69], who said that intervention models will help focus the factors related to couple conflicts to avoid damage that has an impact on the family at the expense of their psychological, physical and labour well-being.

As can be observed, some indicators were isolated in this study to provide guidelines for the psychological intervention in people with couple problems.

5. Limitations

One of the main limitations was the small size of the sample, hence the use of psychometric indexes and cutoff points from the original instruments that were validated for the Mexican population, which limits the generalisation of the results.

Another limitation was that it only measured perceived violence and not exerted violence; in a population that suffers from exerted violence, the profiles will probably differ. One further limitation is that it is a nonprobability sample, and no generalisations can be made, for the results only can show risk indicators for populations with similar characteristics.

It should be noted that another limitation is that it was not a couple study; these results are from women and men with and without marital satisfaction but who were worked with independently. For future research, it would be important to carry out a study of dependent samples where the wife/husband pairing is used.

6. Conclusions

In this study, marital dissatisfaction is 14.5% higher in women; however, generalisations cannot be made, since this study was carried out on a non-random sample in a population with particular characteristics.

The violence perceived from the partner is the same in both groups with marital dissatisfaction.

Marital dissatisfaction is related to submissive characteristics in both sexes.

A decrease in self-esteem is a factor related to couple conflicts.

The type of coping that most contributes to marital dissatisfaction in both sexes is escape/avoidance.

The generation of indicators in different populations by isolating factors that explain the complexity of couple conflicts with no gender biases will contribute to the creation of psychological intervention strategies with greater specificity to avoid the worsening of these conflicts that affect not only both members of the couple but also their surroundings. This work is an incursion in couples who have relationship problems. By isolating explanatory factors, other aspects must be explored in different populations to gain a better understanding of the complexity of couple dynamics.

Author Contributions: Conceptualization, C.S. and C.M.; methodology, C.S.; validation, C.M.; formal analysis, C.S.; investigation, C.S. and C.M.; data curation, C.M.; writing—original draft preparation, C.S.; writing—review and editing, C.S. and C.M.; visualization, C.M.; supervision, C.S.; project administration, C.S. and C.M. All authors have read and agreed to the published version of the manuscript.

Funding: This research received no external funding.

Institutional Review Board Statement: The study was conducted in accordance with the Declaration of Helsinki. This protocol was approved by the research and ethics committees of the National Institute of Perinatology (Protocol number 212250-3110-10810-02-16) and was approved on 17 October 2019.

Informed Consent Statement: Informed consent was obtained from all subjects involved in the study.

Data Availability Statement: The link to the database is added to be consulted https://drive.google.com/file/d/1ndizrROn3jB23Xoi0yRWvH-60aRgLfns/view?usp=sharing (accessed on 24 April 2023).

Acknowledgments: We thank the National Institute of Perinatology for the facilities for this study.

Conflicts of Interest: The authors declare no conflict of interest.

References

1. Ocampo, J. La Elección y Satisfacción en la Relación de Pareja. Master's Thesis, Facultad de Ciencias de la Conducta, UAEM, Toluca, Mexico, 2007.
2. Valdez, J.; Sánchez, G.; Bastida, R.; González, N.; Aguilar, Y. Significado y función del amor como estrategia de sobrevivencia. In *Aportaciones Actuales de la Psicología Social*; AMEPSO: Mexico City, Mexico, 2012; Volume 1, pp. 244–248.
3. Rivera, S.; Díaz-Loving, R. *La Cultura del Poder en la Pareja*; Miguel Ángel Porrúa: Mexico City, Mexico, 2002.
4. Arias-Galicia, F. La escala de satisfacción marital: Análisis de su confiabilidad y validez en una muestra de supervisores mexicanos. *Rev. Interam. Psicol.* **2003**, *37*, 67–92. Available online: https://www.redalyc.org/artículo.oa?id=28437105 (accessed on 24 April 2023).
5. Díaz-Loving, R.; Rivera, S.; Verde, A.; Villanueva, G.; López, C. Valores y manejo del conflicto como determinantes del funcionamiento familiar. *Psicol. Soc. Méx.* **2012**, *XIV*, 725–731.
6. Hurtado, F.; Ciscar, C.; Rubio, M. El conflicto de pareja como variable asociada a la violencia de género contra la mujer: Consecuencias sobre la salud sexual y mental. *Rev. Psicopatol. Psicol. Clín.* **2004**, *9*, 49–64. [CrossRef]
7. Fincham, E.; Hall, J. Parenting and the marital relationship. In *Parenting: An Ecological Perspective*; Lawrence Erlbaum Associates: Mahwah, NJ, USA, 2005; pp. 203–374.
8. Blásquez, M.; Moreno, J.; García, M. La Competencia Emocional Como Recurso Inhibidor Para la Penetración del Maltrato Psicológico en la Pareja. *Salud Ment.* **2012**, *35*, 287–296.
9. Nina, R. El Estudio del Matrimonio desde la Psicología Social. *Rev. Psicol. Soc. Personal.* **2013**, *XXIX*, 59–78.
10. Villegas, M.; Mallor, P. La Dimensión Estructural y Evolutiva en las Relaciones de Pareja. *Ed. UNED* **2012**, *9*, 97–109. Available online: http://www.redalyc.org/articulo.oa?id=344030770009 (accessed on 24 April 2023).
11. Díaz-Loving, R.; Rivera, S.; Velasco, P.; Villanueva, B.; López, B.; Herrera, O. Funcionamiento familiar y satisfacción marital. *Psicol. Soc. Méx.* **2010**, *XV*, 175–182.
12. Flores-Galaz, M.M. Comunicación y Conflicto:¿Que Tanto Importan en la Satisfacción Marital? *Acta Investig. Psicol.* **2011**, *1*, 216–233. Available online: https://www.redalyc.org/articulo.oa?id=358933579003 (accessed on 24 April 2023). [CrossRef]
13. Torres, M. *La Violencia en Casa*; Paidós: Mexico City, Mexico, 2005.

14. Sánchez, M.; del Pilar, M.; Rangel, B.; Adrian; Gómez, P.; Rafael; Méndez, G.; Mirna. Severidad de la violencia de pareja y reacciones emocionales en mujeres. *Psicumex* **2022**, *12*, e400. [CrossRef]
15. Piccinini, A.; Bailo, P.; Barbara, G.; Miozzo, M.; Tabano, S.; Colapietro, P.; Farè, C.; Sirchia, S.M.; Battaglioli, E.; Bertuccio, P.; et al. Violence against Women and Stress-Related Disorders: Seeking for Associated Epigenetic Signatures, a Pilot Study. *Healthcare* **2023**, *11*, 173. [CrossRef]
16. Ocampo y Amar. Violencia de Pareja, las Caras del Fenómeno. *Rev. Salud Uninorte* **2011**, *27*, 108–123. Available online: http://www.scielo.org.co/scielo.php?script=sci_arttext&pid=S0120-55522011000100011&lng=en&tlng=es (accessed on 24 April 2023).
17. Gracia, E. *Las Víctimas Invisibles de la Violencia Familiar: El Extraño Iceberg de la Violencia Doméstica*; Paidós: Barcelona, Spain, 2002.
18. Navarro, N.; Salguero, A.; Torres, L.E.; Figueroa, J.G. Voces silenciadas: Hombres que viven violencia en la relación de pareja. *Rev. Estud. Género Ventana* **2019**, *6*, 136–172. [CrossRef]
19. Amor, P.; Echeburúa, E.; Loinaz, I. ¿Se Puede Establecer una Clasificación Tipológica de los Hombres Violentos Contra su Pareja? *Int. J. Clin. Health Psychol.* **2009**, *9*, 519–539. Available online: http://www.redalyc.org/artículo.oa?id=33712038010 (accessed on 24 April 2023).
20. Aroca, C.; Garrido, V. La máscara del amor. Programa de prevención de la violencia en la pareja. In *Manual de Conocimientos del Profesorado*; Serrano Villalba, C., Ed.; DATOS.BNE.ES: Valencia, Spain, 2005.
21. Aroca, C.; Lorenzo, M.; Miró, C. La violencia filio-parental: Un análisis de sus claves. *Anal. Psicol.* **2014**, *30*, 157–170. [CrossRef]
22. García, M. Una Visión Cultural de las Dimensiones y Correlatos de la Violencia en la Relación de Pareja. Bachelor's Thesis, Facultad de Psicología, UNAM, Mexico City, Mexico, 2002.
23. Ramos, L.; Saltijeral, M. ¿Violencia Episódica o Terrorismo Íntimo? Una Propuesta Exploratoria Para Clasificar la Violencia Contra la Mujer en las Relaciones de Pareja. *Salud Ment.* **2008**, *31*, 469–478. Available online: http://www.scielo.org.mx/scielo.php?script=sci_arttext&pid=S0185-33252008000600007&lng=es&tlng=es (accessed on 24 April 2023).
24. Burgos, D.; Canaval, G.; Tobo, N.; Bernal, P.; Humphreys. Violencia de Pareja en Mujeres de la Comunidad Tipos y Severidad. *Rev. Salud Públ.* **2012**, *14*, 77–89. Available online: http://bit.ly/2rww.DLG (accessed on 24 April 2023).
25. Morales, A.; Alonso, M.; López, K. Violencia de Género y Autoestima de las Mujeres de la Ciudad de Puebla. *Rev. Sanid. Mil. Méx.* **2011**, *65*, 48–52. Available online: htpp://bit.ly/2q7TcWV (accessed on 24 April 2023).
26. Juárez, C.; Valdez, R.; Hernández, D. La Percepción del Apoyo Social en Mujeres con Experiencia de Violencia Conyugal. *Salud Ment.* **2005**, *28*, 66–73.
27. Tuesca, R.; Borda, M. Violencia Física Marital en Barranquilla (Colombia): Prevalencia y Factores de Riesgo. *Gac. Sanit.* **2003**, *17*, 302–308. Available online: http://scielo.isciii.es/scielo.php?script=sci_arttext&pid=S0213-91112003000400008&lng=es&tlng=es (accessed on 24 April 2023). [CrossRef]
28. Cienfuegos, Y.I. Medición de la violencia en las relaciones de pareja. *Culturales* **2021**, *9*, e544. [CrossRef]
29. Mapayi, B.; Makanjuola, R.O.A.; Mosaku, S.K.; Adewuya, O.A.; Afolabi, O.; Aloba, O.O.; Akinsulore, A. Impact of intimate partner violence on anxiety and depression amongst women in Ile-Ife, Nigeria. *Arch. Women's Ment. Health* **2013**, *16*, 11–18. [CrossRef] [PubMed]
30. Gage, A.J.; Thomas, N.J. Women's Work, Gender Roles, and Intimate Partner Violence in Nigeria. *Arch. Sex. Behav.* **2017**, *46*, 1923–1938. [CrossRef] [PubMed]
31. Aizer, A. The Gender Wage Gap and Domestic Violence. *Am. Econ. Rev.* **2010**, *100*, 1847–1859. [CrossRef] [PubMed]
32. Rocha, S.T. Socialización y Cultura: El Impacto de la Diferenciación Entre los Sexos. Ph.D. Thesis, Facultad de Psicología, Universidad Nacional Autónoma de México, Mexico City, Mexico, 2004.
33. Díaz Loving, R.; Rocha, T.; Rivera, S. *La Instrumentalidad y Expresividad Desde una Perspectiva Psico-Socio-Cultural*; Miguel Ángel Porrúa: Mexico City, Mexico, 2007.
34. Stoller, R. *Sex and Gender*; Science House: Raleigh, NC, USA, 1968.
35. Herrera, P. Rol de Género y Funcionamiento Familiar. *Rev. Cubana Méd. Género Integr.* **2000**, *16*, 568–573. Available online: http://scielo.sld.cu/scielo.php?script=sci_arttext&pid=S0864-21252000000600008&lng=es&tlng=es (accessed on 24 April 2023).
36. Shechory, M.; Ziv, R. Relationships between Gender Role Attitudes, Role Division, and Perception of Equity among Heterosexual, Gay and Lesbian Couples. *Sex Roles* **2007**, *56*, 629–638. [CrossRef]
37. Sanchez, D.T.; Phelan, J.E.; Moss-Racusin, C.A.; Good, J.J. The Gender Role Motivation Model of Women's Sexually Submissive Behavior and Satisfaction in Heterosexual Couples. *Personal. Soc. Psychol. Bull.* **2012**, *38*, 528–539. [CrossRef] [PubMed]
38. Cañete, M.; Reis, E.; Moleiro, C. The roles of culture, gender norms, and sexual orientation in intimate partner violence: Psychosocial variables associated with IPV in a Portuguese sample. *Couple Fam. Psychol. Res. Pract.* **2022**. Advance online publication. [CrossRef]
39. Cazés, D. La dimensión social del género: Posibilidad de vida para mujeres y hombres en el patriarcado. In *Antología de la Sexualidad Humana I*; Pérez, E.C., Ed.; Porrúa: Jalisco, Mexico, 2002; pp. 335–387.
40. Cardenal, V. *El Autoconcepto y la Autoestima en el Desarrollo de la Madurez Personal*; Ediciones Aljibe: Archidona, Spain, 1999.
41. Nava, V.; Onofre, D.; Báez, F. Autoestima, violencia de pareja y conducta sexual en mujeres indígenas. *Enferm. Univ.* **2017**, *14*, 162–169. [CrossRef]

42. Murray, S.L.; Rose, P.; Bellavia, G.M.; Holmes, J.G.; Kusche, A.G. When rejection stings: How self-esteem constrains relationship-enhancement processes. *J. Personal. Soc. Psychol.* **2002**, *83*, 556–573. [CrossRef]
43. Erol, R.; Orth, U. Self-Esteem and the Quality of Romantic Relationships. *Eur. Psychol.* **2017**, *21*, 274–283. [CrossRef]
44. Aguilar, R.J.; Nightingale, N.N. The impact of specific battering experiences on the self-esteem of abused women. *J. Fam. Viol.* **1994**, *9*, 35–45. [CrossRef]
45. González, B.; Montoya, C.; Casullo, M.; Bernabéu, V. Relación Entre Estilos y Estrategias de Afrontamiento y Bienestar Psicológico en Adolescentes. *Psiocothema* **2002**, *14*, 363–368. Available online: http://www.redalyc.org/articulo.oa?id=72714227 (accessed on 24 April 2023).
46. Escriba, A.; Bernabé, M. Estrategias de Afrontamiento Ante el Estrés y Fuentes de Recompensa Profesional en Médicos Especialistas de la Comunidad Valenciana: Un Estudio con Entrevistas Semiestructuradas. *Rev. Esp. Salud Públ.* **2002**, *5*, 595–604. Available online: http://scielo.isciii.es/scielo.php?script=sci_arttext&pid=S1135-57272002000500019&lng=es&ting=es (accessed on 24 April 2023). [CrossRef]
47. Góngora, C.; Reyes, L. La estructura de los estilos de enfrentamiento: Rasgo y estado en un ecosistema tradicional mexicano. *Rev. Son. Psicol.* **1999**, *13*, 3–14.
48. Góngora, C. El Enfrentamiento a los Problemas y el Papel del Control: Una Visión Etnopsicológica en un Ecosistema con Tradición. Ph.D. Thesis, UNAM, Mexico City, Mexico, 2000.
49. Plata, M.; Castillo, O.; Guevara, L. Evaluación de afrontamiento, depresión y ansiedad e incapacidad funcional en pacientes con dolor crónico. *Rev. Mex. Anestesiol.* **2004**, *27*, 16–23.
50. Lazarus, R.; Folkman, S. *Estrés y Procesos Cognitivos*; Ediciones Roca: Barcelona, Spain, 1991.
51. Sayem, A.; Begum, H.; Moneesha, S. Women's attitudes towards formal and informal support-seeking coping strategies aganist intimate partner violence. *J. Homepage.* **2013**, *58*, 270–286. [CrossRef]
52. Puente-Martínez, A.; Ubillos-Landa, S.; Páez-Rovira, D. Problem-Focused Coping Strategies Used by Victims of Gender Violence Across the Stages of Change. *J. Homepage.* **2021**, *28*, 3331–3351. [CrossRef] [PubMed]
53. Cañetas, E.; Rivera, S.; Díaz-Loving, R. Desarrollo de un instrumento de satisfacción marital (IMUSA). *Psicol. Soc. Méx.* **2000**, *VIII*, 266–274.
54. Cienfuegos, J. Evaluación del Conflicto Satisfacción Marital y Apoyo Social en Mujeres Violentadas: Un Estudio Comparativo. Bachelor's Thesis, UNAM, Mexico City, Mexico, 2004.
55. Lara, A. *Inventario Masculinidad y Femineidad*; El Manual Moderno: Mexico City, Mexico, 1993.
56. Lara, C.; Verduzco, M.; Acevedo, M.; Cortés, J. Validez y Confiabilidad del Inventario de Autoestima de Coopersmith Para adultos, en Población Mexicana. *Rev. Latinoam. Psicol.* **1993**, *25*, 247–255. Available online: http://www.redalyc.org/articulo.oa?id=80525207 (accessed on 24 April 2023).
57. Zavala, L.; Rivas, R.; Andrade, P.; Reidl, L. Validación del Instrumento de Estilos de Enfrentamiento de Lazarus y Folkman en adultos de la Ciudad de México. *Rev. Intercont. Psicol. Educ.* **2008**, *2*, 159–182. Available online: http://www.redalyc.org/articulo.oa?id=80212387009 (accessed on 24 April 2023).
58. Moral, J.; López, F.; Díaz-Loving, R.; Cienfuegos, Y. Diferencias de Género en Afrontamiento y Violencia en la Pareja. *Rev. CES Psicol.* **2011**, *4*, 29–46. Available online: http://www.redalyc.org/articulo.oa?id=423539528004 (accessed on 24 April 2023).
59. Medina, M.E.; Riquer, F.; Castro, P.R. *Volencia de Género en las Parejas Mexicanas: Resultados de la Encuesta Nacional Sobre la Dinámica de las Relaciones en los Hogares*; Centro Regional de Investigaciones Multidisciplinarias/UNAM: Mexico City, Mexico, 2006; Available online: http://bibliotecavirtual.clacso.org.ar/Mexico/crim-unam/20100428121317/Violencia_parejas.pdf (accessed on 24 April 2023).
60. Rodríguez-Hernández, R.; Esquivel-Santoveña, E.E. Prevalencia y factores asociados con la violencia de pareja en las adultas mayores mexicanas. *Salud Colect.* **2020**, *16*, e2600. [CrossRef]
61. Vizcarra, B.; Póo, M. Violencia de pareja en estudiantes universitarios del sur de Chile. *Univ. Psychol.* **2011**, *10*, 89–98. [CrossRef]
62. Castro, R.; Casique, I. Violencia de pareja contra las mujeres en México: Una comparación entre encuestas recientes. *Notas Poblac.* **2005**, *35*, 35–61.
63. Cervantes, C.; Ramos, L.; Saltijeral, M. Frecuencia y dimensiones de la violencia emocional contra la mujer por parte del compañero íntimo. Violencia contra las mujeres en contextos urbanos y rurales. In *El Colegio de México/Programa Interdisciplinario de Estudios de la Mujer*; Torres, E.M., Ed.; El Colegio de Mexico: Mexico City, Mexico, 2004; pp. 239–270.
64. Aiquipa, J. Dependencia Emocional en Mujeres Víctimas de Violencia de Pareja. *Rev. Psicol.* **2015**, *33*, 412–437. Available online: http://pepsic.bvsalud.org/pdf/rp/v33n2/a07v33n2.pdf (accessed on 24 April 2023). [CrossRef]
65. Echeburúa, E.; Amor, P.; de Corral, P. Hombres Violentos Contra la Pareja: Trastornos Mentales y Perfiles Psicológicos. *Pensam. Psicológico* **2009**, *6*, 27–36. Available online: http://www.redalyc.org/artículo.oa?id=80112469003 (accessed on 24 April 2023).
66. Méndez, M.; García, M. Relación Entre las Estrategias de Manejo del Conflicto y la Percepción de la Violencia Situacional en la Pareja. *Rev. Colomb. Psicol.* **2015**, *24*, 99–111. Available online: http://www.redalyc.org/articulo.oa?id=80438019007(65) (accessed on 24 April 2023). [CrossRef]
67. Moral, J.; López, F. Modelo recursivo de reacción violenta en parejas válido para ambos sexos. *Boletín Psicol.* **2012**, *105*, 61–74.

68. MacLean, D.; Kermode, S. A study of the relationship between quality of life, health and self-esteem. *Aust. J. Adv. Nurs.* **2001**, *19*, 33–40.
69. Santelices, M.; Guzmán, M.; Garrido, L. Apego y Psicopatología: Estudio Comparativo de los Estilos de Apego en Adultos con y sin Sintomatología Ansioso-Depresivo. *Rev. Argent. Clín. Psicol.* **2011**, *XX*, 49–55. Available online: http://www.redalyc.org/articulo.oa?id=281921807004 (accessed on 24 April 2023).

Disclaimer/Publisher's Note: The statements, opinions and data contained in all publications are solely those of the individual author(s) and contributor(s) and not of MDPI and/or the editor(s). MDPI and/or the editor(s) disclaim responsibility for any injury to people or property resulting from any ideas, methods, instructions or products referred to in the content.

MDPI
St. Alban-Anlage 66
4052 Basel
Switzerland
www.mdpi.com

Healthcare Editorial Office
E-mail: healthcare@mdpi.com
www.mdpi.com/journal/healthcare

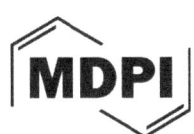

Disclaimer/Publisher's Note: The statements, opinions and data contained in all publications are solely those of the individual author(s) and contributor(s) and not of MDPI and/or the editor(s). MDPI and/or the editor(s) disclaim responsibility for any injury to people or property resulting from any ideas, methods, instructions or products referred to in the content.

www.ingramcontent.com/pod-product-compliance
Lightning Source LLC
LaVergne TN
LVHW070624100526
838202LV00012B/718